Mastering Menopause

By

Igor Klibanov

Table of Contents

- When fat gain during menopause might actually be a good thing and when it isn't.
- What really happens to your metabolism during menopause.
- The myth of a universally optimal hormone level.
- Why is weight gained specifically around the middle?

- How many calories should you eat if you want to lose weight? Surprise: it might be more than you think.
- Caffeine and hot flashes.
- What foods to eat to reduce menopausal symptoms.
- An alcoholic beverage that's surprisingly good for menopausal symptoms (no, not red wine).
- Menopause, bones and calcium – how much calcium do you really need?
- How to maintain lean muscle during and after menopause.

- The 4 biggest reasons why diets fail (and they're not nutritional)
- A simple technique to help you distinguish between hunger and emotional eating.
- What is mindful eating, and how do you do it?
- How to plan your meals properly – while including your favourite "cheat meals."
- How to address stress – without eating foods you know you shouldn't.
- How to design your environment to make fat loss effortless.

- Why information isn't motivation, and what's actually required for long-term behavior change.
- 4 questions you need to ask yourself to boost your motivation.
- Behavior goals vs. outcome goals – which one should you focus on?
- Why making small changes can lead to big results.
- Why trying to make big changes can lead to failure.
- The mentality you need to apply to healthy eating that will ensure you don't fall off the bandwagon.

- Should postmenopausal women exercise differently than premenopausal women?

- How does exercise affect the hormone levels of postmenopausal women?
- What's the least amount of cardio you can do and still improve your endurance?
- Sample strength training workout.
- Sample cardio workout.

- Why do women experience more injuries in the 10 years before and after menopause?
- How estrogen levels affect your injury risk.
- How progesterone levels affect your injury risk.
- How testosterone levels affect your injury risk.

- 2 myths about supplements.
- 3 reasons why I REALLY like supplements.
- 4 effective supplements to reduce menopausal symptoms.
- 2 ineffective ingredients for menopause – even though they're often included in menopause supplements.
- 7 unproven supplements for menopause.
- How to combine supplements safely.
- Why ineffective and unproven ingredients are often included in menopause supplements.

- A common sleep condition that gets even more common during and after menopause.
- A simple technique used for anxiety – that works to improve sleep as well.
- One of the most powerful methods of normalizing your sleep during and after menopause.

- How Julie's body changed during menopause.
- The exercise strategies that she used to lower her blood pressure, get rid of joint pain and lose weight.
- The nutritional strategies that she used.
- The results she achieved.
- The obstacles Julie faced along the way.
- How her life is different today.

- The exercise strategies that she used.
- The nutritional strategies that she used.
- The results she achieved.
- How her life is different today.

Acknowledgements

Barbara is a veterinarian of over 30 years' experience, who has written a book of her own: *Whiskers to Tail – Health Conditions of Dogs and Cats.*

Cristina met Igor at one of his workshops about health and exercising in 2014, after she turned 50. After subscribing to his newsletter and attending several other seminars of his over the years, she decided to join his exercise training program at Fitness Solutions Plus in Markham, Ontario in order to improve her physical endurance and overall health. Part of his program is undergoing the Poliquin hormone body fat profile and completing a comprehensive health assessment covering the diet, lifestyle, general and chronic health which help to personalize the physical training and lifestyle journey back to health. At various points in time over the years, Cristina has worked with 3 of Igor's personal trainers who all share his vision and knowledge.

Disha Alam is a friend who practices as a hospitalist midwife at McMaster Children's Hospital. She's also a part-time lecturer in the midwifery program at Toronto Metropolitan University. She completed her Masters in Health Administration.

Eden Tsafaroff works as a healthcare regulator and has a background in clinical investigations and health and safety. She is interested in the motivation behind behaviours that lead to complaints and finds resolution of a case to be very rewarding. In her free time, Eden enjoys creative writing and has a children's book on Kindle (Analu and her Rainbow Lollipop).

George Stavrou is both a friend and former client who has decades of experience in the fitness/nutrition industry, and now, runs a comprehensive online health program called "The Stavrou Method." You can check it out by visiting https:// thestavroumethod.com.

Heather Skoll is a Certified Kripalu Yoga Teacher and Certified Rubenfeld Synergist. Heather has a few years of experience in menopause and has been through some of the very physical challenges and changes as described in Igor's book. Heather is thrilled that Igor's book will be available to help her inform her adapted chair yoga clients, and hopefully millions of others.

Ingrid Trulsen's foray into fitness began at an early age participating in outdoor activities with her family all year long. By 1980 she became interested in "aerobics", Jane Fonda, and the "20 Min Workout". Her first official cardio sessions were at home using a vinyl record and a booklet with the moves - all performed to the theme song from the TV show Dallas!

Later on, at the age of 43, she became a personal trainer/fitness instructor in downtown Toronto. To this day at the age of 57, Ingrid still regularly incorporates handstands and gymnastic headstands into her workouts. As a self-proclaimed die-hard optimist, her motto is "never give up!"

Ingrid currently lives and works in Montréal, QC.

Kara Crumb has an honours bachelor of kinesiology from Lakehead University and is currently pursuing her masters degree in kinesiology at Lakehead. Kara is a personal trainer at Body Fit health club in Uxbridge and is physiotherapy assistant doing home visits throughout southern Ontario. Kara enjoys the gym, hiking, hanging out with friends and petting all the cute animals.

Melissa McNally is a Registered Kinesiologist with over 5 years experience in working with people who have chronic disease. She enjoys helping others improve their quality of life. As well, she enjoys learning and was excited to be a part of this book.

Polina Avraham is an optimistic go getter. Having lived in Kazakhstan and Israel, Polina lives now with her busy family (husband, two teenagers and two big dogs) in the Greater Toronto Area, Ontario, Canada. She works in the insurance industry.

She loves to integrate physical activity in her daily routine. A run, hike in the woods, walking dogs, Zumba or yoga class in a nearby studio, bicycle ride, lifting weights or cardio training session - one of those always makes its way into her daily schedule.

When it is time to relax, a massage therapy session, coffee in a local shop, or Epsom salt bath are the preferred ways to treat herself to unwind from the noise of the day.

She describes herself as a kind, caring, happy and very health-conscious individual, who approaches life with endless optimism and a can-do attitude.

Rekha Kulshreshtha is a management consultant with over 30 years of experience in helping organizations transform with a focus on people, processes, and technology. After more than 25 years working for a large multinational technology company, she founded RK Transformation Consulting Services and continues to support clients in their transformation journeys. She has been a regular client for 4 years and was happy to contribute her input to this book.

Chapter 1

Introduction

You're probably holding this book for one of 3 reasons:

- Menopause is on the horizon for you, and you want to know what to expect once it hits. You've heard some things, and you want to be proactive about it once you hit menopause.
- You're knee-deep in menopause and are experiencing some changes that you're not so fond of, like weight gain, hot flashes, fatigue, brain fog, and others. You want to know how to manage all these symptoms using exercise, nutrition and supplements.
- Menopause is in the rearview mirror for you, but you're still experiencing symptoms or want to change the negative effects it's had on your body.

Regardless of which category you fit into, there's something here for you. This book is all about how to manage menopausal symptoms and health consequences using exercise, nutrition and supplements.

What Can You Expect?

You might have a lot of questions about menopause, like:

- How can I reduce my hot flashes?
- How can I manage my mood swings?
- How can I improve my energy levels?

- Is it possible to experience a seamless menopause with just lifestyle interventions?

...and the big one: how do I lose weight after menopause? The things that used to work for me in my 20s and 30s no longer work for me in my 40s, 50s, 60s and beyond. And why did the fat shift from my buns and thighs to my belly?

To answer your questions:

To reduce the symptoms of menopause, follow the advice in this book. Either just the bits and pieces that are easy for you, or the whole thing. Of course, you'll get the greatest, fastest, and most long-lasting reductions if you follow everything. But even if you can't or don't want to, that's fine. Any single strategy here can improve your menopause experience. And every little bit counts.

For the menopause diet, you'll learn how to eat the foods you love, while still being able to lose weight (if you need to lose weight – you'll learn later on). You'll even learn about a common alcoholic beverage that can improve your menopausal symptoms (no, it's not red wine). I'll bet you didn't think you'd read about that in a nutrition book. I guess I had to compensate in some way for being a guy who's writing this book.

Do supplements work? The only thing I can guarantee is this: nothing works for 100% of the people, 100% of the time. Not medications, not surgery, not exercise, not supplements. However, I will tell you about several supplements that have the most potent effects on menopausal symptoms (and we'll differentiate between the different types of symptoms, from hot flashes to the psychological ones), with minimal-to-no side effects. And I'll also tell you which supplements are not worth your money.

Sound like a good deal? Good. I want you to succeed at this.

This book is aimed to satisfy both the geek, who wants to know the mechanisms and the science behind all the recommendations, as well as the "give me the bottom line" straight shooter. Want the bottom line without any of the science? Flip to the conclusion chapter, and you'll find your menopause exercise, nutrition and supplementation program in an accessible spot, where you can consume it in under 5 minutes – without the scientific explanations.

I'm sure my skeptical readers might wonder "Where is this information coming from?" I'll tell you.

I'm a personal trainer. I train clients who have various conditions, like high blood pressure, arthritis, osteoporosis, and others. One of the most common reasons that clients come to me is menopause. And I hate not being able to get results with my clients. So as soon as I have a client with an issue that I know about generally, but maybe not specifically, I get to work. I geek out on the medical research about that topic. Not mainstream books or YouTube videos – but studies. Ideally, double-blind, placebo-controlled studies.

Then I start implementing what I've learned with my clients, to check whether the theory matches the practice. If it does, I then try it with additional clients who have the same issue. Then, I write about my findings in my blog (www. FitnessSolutionsPlus.ca/blog). Then I take on even more clients with this condition, after they read those blogs. Eventually, by the time I get to writing a book about the topic, my team and I have helped dozens of people with the issue you're reading about directly, in one-on-one settings and hundreds or even thousands through my blogs and books indirectly.

But just as it's important to know what we'll cover, it's just as important to know what we won't cover. Here's what will **not** be covered in this book:

- Cancer
- Skin
- Sexual function
- Hormone replacement therapy

Again, I want my book to come from both the scientific theory, as well as my practical experience. Not just one or the other. As a personal trainer, I never get clients who want improvements in their cancer outcomes, skin care or sexual function. That's not what people go to most personal trainers for. But my menopausal clients do come to me for help with weight loss, toning and reduction of symptoms. So I'll speak to what I know and have worked with. What I don't know or haven't worked with, I'll leave for other qualified professionals and authors to discuss.

And hey, if we're going to spend the next few hours together, why don't we get better acquainted?

Let me introduce myself.

I'm Igor. Nice to meet ya.

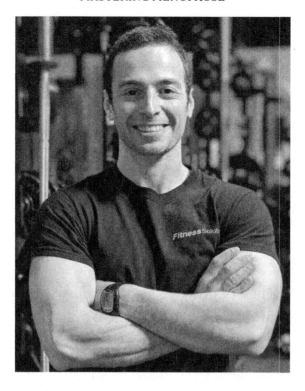

I have a degree in kinesiology and health science, as well as multiple diplomas in clinical nutrition. I was selected as one of the top 5 personal trainers in Toronto by the Metro News newspaper, written 11 other books, as well as over 500 articles (at the time of this writing) on my blog (FitnessSolutionsPlus.ca/blog). I've been hired by some of Canada's largest corporations to speak on topics like how to reverse chronic conditions and have done approximately 50 speaking engagements per year for the last 12 years.

So, you might ask "Why is a personal trainer writing about menopause?" Because unlike most personal trainers, who work with athletes, models and bodybuilders, my specialty is "the big 4 plus 1." The "big 4", being:

- High blood pressure
- Type 2 diabetes
- Osteoporosis
- Osteoarthritis

The "plus 1" is menopause.

I'll admit that I thought long and hard about writing a book on menopause. After all – I'm a man. I'll never have it, so do I really have any credibility to be writing about it? While I don't have any personal credibility, I have a lot of professional credibility. My team and I have helped hundreds of menopausal and postmenopausal clients lose weight and improve their menopausal symptoms. Two of those clients are featured in the last two chapters of this book.

I've read a lot of books on menopause. But when I dove into the medical literature, I learned so many more interesting, practical, and effective strategies to lose weight, and manage menopausal symptoms. Once my team and I started implementing those strategies with clients, and getting great results, I thought it was too good not to share. Much of this information, I've never seen in other books on menopause. My team and I are limited by how many clients we can train and give our attention to, but a book can go anywhere in the world. So I hope that the information in this book will help you as well.

I LOOOOOVVVEEEE hearing success stories. I want to hear yours. So after you've implemented what's in this book, I want to hear from you. Email me and let me know how you did. My email is Igor@TorontoFitnessOnline.com.

Additionally, if you like what you read in this book, and want to stay in touch, I have a free newsletter. You can sign up for it by visiting www.Mastering-Menopause.com.

Chapter 2

9 Menopause Myths That Are Harming Your Health

There are plenty of myths about menopause. Some of them, you might actually believe. Lucky for you that you're reading this book, because in this chapter, we'll bust 9 of the most common myths about menopause, and answer a couple of frequently asked questions.

Before we jump in, let's just give some definitions of common terms:

- Premenopause: all the years from birth until you stop having periods.
- Perimenopause: the transition to menopause. This is when hormone levels drop, periods become more irregular, until you stop having periods. This could be as long as 10 years.
- Menopause: one year since your last period.
- Postmenopause: all the years after menopause.

  With those definitions out of the way, let's start mythbusting. In no particular order:

Myth #1: All Women Gain Weight During and After Menopause

Very often, is we're in a certain undesirable position, we think that others are as well. We think our situation is universal. After all, misery loves company.

But **not all women gain weight during menopause**.

In one study[91], 591 premenopausal women were recruited who were expected to be menopausal or postmenopausal over the next 5 years.

After 5 years, of the 591 women, 109 women (18%) actually lost 3% of their body weight. 255 women (43%) maintained their weight. And 227 women (39%) gained weight.

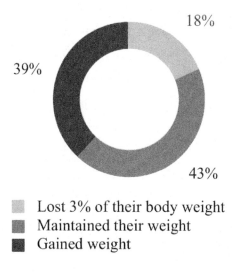

18%

39%

43%

 Lost 3% of their body weight
 Maintained their weight
 Gained weight

In another study[69] of 497 women, 29% of them maintained their weight during and after menopause. 12% of them lost weight and 59% gained weight.

The overall message is that the number of women who gain weight during and after menopause varies study by study, but not all women gain weight during and after menopause. Some do and some don't. What is it that differentiates those who do, and those who don't? I'll cover that in myth #7. Keep reading 😊

Myth #2: Weight Gain in Menopause is Bad

We're often told that weight gain is bad, as a blanket statement. But that's not true for a lot of people who gain weight. People who were underweight to begin with, and gain weight, experience a healthy weight gain. Likewise, women who had an ideal BMI (body mass index – that's your weight in kg, divided by your height in meters squared. Stated another way, that's kg/m²) before menopause actually **experience improvements in health and vitality when they go from a "normal" BMI (which is 18.5-24.9) to slightly overweight** (a BMI of 25.0-29.9). This doesn't apply to women who were overweight and became obese (BMI >30).

$$\text{BMI} = \frac{\text{weight}_{kg}}{\text{height}_{m}^{2}}$$

Wait, what? Why is a personal trainer is saying that weight gain is healthy post menopause? Surely, he must mean from muscle? No, I don't. Actual **body fat gain during and after menopause is a good thing**. But don't take my word for it. Here's some research:

In one study[84] of 6030 people, lean menopausal women (who had a BMI of under 25) who gained weight actually had a **65% reduction in their risk of all-cause mortality** (risk of dying for any reason – heart disease, cancer, dementia, etc.). How much weight, you ask? As much as 22 lbs. (10 kg). The same study showed that on the other hand, when premenopausal women gain weight, their risk of all-cause mortality rises by 5%.

One systematic review[9] showed that **weight loss in postmenopausal women did not reduce the risk of heart disease**. In other words, some postmenopausal women who exercised and improved their nutrition lost weight, and others didn't. Regardless of whether weight was lost, there was a reduction in the risk of heart disease. So it's not the weight loss that improved it, but rather, improved exercise and nutrition – even if it didn't lead to weight loss.

To summarize the research, weight gain in premenopausal women who were of normal weight to begin with is not good. But weight gain in postmenopausal women who were of normal weight and became slightly overweight *is* good. Weight gain in postmenopausal women who were of normal weight or even overweight and became obese is not good either.

Ain't that interesting?

Are you wondering why weight gain (and again, we're talking about fat gain, not muscle) has such a positive effect on disease risk in postmenopausal women?

Estrogen. Besides age, one of the reasons that younger women have lower rates of heart disease compared to older women is that they have higher estrogen levels.

Estrogen

OH

HO

Before menopause, the **3 organs that make estrogen are the ovaries, adrenal glands and body fat**. After menopause, the ovaries don't do the job anymore, so most of the estrogen is made by the adrenal glands and body fat. So **women who do gain body fat also have more estrogen** (and we used to think that body fat was just passive tissue. We now that that it isn't. Body fat is a hormone-secreting organ in its own right. And it's responsible in the production of more than just estrogen, but that's a discussion for another time), and all the benefits that come with more estrogen, like:

- Better skin quality
- Better mood
- Better sleep
- Better focus
- Less brain fog,

and the biggie: a 65% lower risk of all-cause mortality. The term "all-cause mortality" means the risk of dying for any reason (heart disease, cancer, dementia, etc.).

How much more estrogen do overweight women have compared to lean women? According to one study[86], about **50% more**.

But what about menopausal symptoms? You might be thinking "Maybe the length of life is longer, but the quality of life is lower." Do women who gain body fat have more menopausal symptoms? If a woman is overweight, her menopausal symptoms aren't any higher than a lean woman. But if a woman is obese, yes, she has worse menopausal symptoms.

In one study[77] of 749 postmenopausal women, they were divided into 3 categories, based on their BMI:

- Group 1 had a BMI under 25 (considered "lean")
- Group 2 had a BMI of 25-29.9 (considered "overweight")
- Group 3 had a BMI of 30 or higher (considered "obese")

Here are the highlights:

- The frequency and severity of symptoms (all menopausal symptoms – not just hot flashes) were almost identical between the lean and overweight women.
- The obese women had 17% more hot flashes compared to the overweight women, and their hot flashes were more severe.
- There was a 14% increase in muscle and joint problems between the overweight and obese women.
- There was a 29% increase in depression between the overweight and obese women.
- There was a 29% increase in sleep problems between the overweight and obese women.
- Twice as many obese women had bladder problems compared to overweight women.

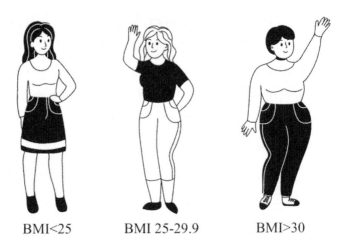

BMI<25   BMI 25-29.9   BMI>30

In essence, the results of numerous studies on fat gain during and after menopause can be summarized as follows: **"Being overweight is advantageous, while being obese is not."**

Does that mean that if you're a lean postmenopausal woman, you should deliberately try to add body fat? Sounds like fun, doesn't it? But no, I wouldn't advise that. So don't get a membership to your local buffet.

As you'll learn in the following myths, **body fat is gained involuntarily**. Likely because the body wants a certain level of estrogen. If you're a lean woman, and you're experiencing minimal to no menopausal symptoms, you don't need to gain body fat. But if you're a lean woman, and you are experiencing menopausal symptoms, try implementing the advice in the rest of this book. If after 3 months, you don't see an improvement, it might actually be time to gain body fat. Although I have no research to back this up, a handful of times, I've told female clients to deliberately gain body fat.

When do I do it? When they meet these criteria:

- They're experiencing estrogen-deficiency symptoms.
- Their body fat is very low (for a woman, below around 15%).

Lastly, before moving on to the next myth, I can feel the savvy, well-informed reader criticizing BMI as a method of assessing body fat. The typical argument against BMI is that **it just takes weight and height into account**. But if someone is very muscular, it'll classify them as overweight/obese, even though they're lean.

I get that. But to counter that point, first of all, **on a population basis, BMI works just fine**. Most of the population doesn't exercise. Second of all, the portion of the population that does exercise isn't doing so with the express intent of gaining maximum muscle. They want to gain a bit of muscle and lose a bit of fat. They're not trying to be Arnold Schwarzenegger. A gain of 4-6 pounds of muscle won't make a difference to BMI. Only a tiny percent of the population (probably under 1% of postmenopausal women) is so muscular where BMI is not a good gauge.

Again, on a population basis, BMI gets the job done. But even then, not in every population. **BMI works well in the Caucasian population**. But what if you're not Caucasian? Here are some general rules[12]:

- East Asian Women (Chinese, Japanese, Korean, etc.) have a higher body fat at the same BMI. For them, obesity doesn't start at a BMI of 30, but rather, 27.
- For East Indian Women, it's the same as East Asian Women, but even more exaggerated. For them, obesity starts at a BMI of 26.

- As for Black people, the relationship between BMI and body fat is complicated. On average, Black people gain more body fat with age, compared to Caucasians, Asians and East Indians. There are also significant differences between African Americans, Jamaicans and Africans. But in almost all Black people body fat percentage is lower at the same BMI compared to Caucasians. So as a rough estimate (this one is my opinion only), for them, obesity starts at a BMI of 31.

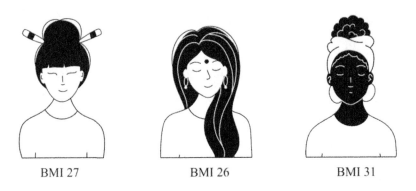

BMI 27   BMI 26   BMI 31

While BMI is good on a population basis, when studying large numbers of people, **on an individual basis, I prefer to use body fat**. It solves the problems with BMI. What's the best way to measure body fat? That's another debate in an of itself. I wrote an entire report on the different methods of body fat testing (like the body fat scale, handheld device, underwater dunking, DEXA scans, calipers, etc.), along with their pros and cons. I've made that report available to you for free at www.Mastering-Menopause.com.

Nonetheless, what are the body fat guidelines that I use with clients? I like to see menopausal and postmenopausal women in the 18-28% body fat range. Above 28%, and we try to reduce it. Below

18%, and we try to either maintain if they're feeling fine or raise their body fat if they're experiencing estrogen-deficiency symptoms.

Now, I get it. When you picked up this book, maybe your biggest reason was to lose weight, and here you are, getting advice like "weight loss may not be advisable." Lots of my clients have beautiful dresses, jeans, and tops that they really like, but are now feeling snug, or they just can't fit into them.

So it's a bit of a psychological battle between what you're used to, and what's healthy at this point in your life.

Myth #3: My Metabolism Slowed Down

The women who gain weight during and after menopause often attribute it to their metabolism slowing down. It makes sense. It's logical, but it's not correct.

It's undeniable that weight is gained. But the reason for that weight gain is largely (but not entirely) misattributed.

There's a concept called "**Total Daily Energy Expenditure**" (or TDEE for short). There are 4 components to TDEE:

- **Basal Metabolic Rate** (BMR): this is how many calories you burn just to stay alive. How much energy it takes to keep your brain working, your blood flowing, your liver/kidney filtering, etc.
- **Thermic Effect of Food** (TEF): you don't absorb 100% of the calories that you eat. You absorb about 90% (although this varies slightly based on the composition of your diet).

So you use 10% of the calories you eat for digestion, absorption and elimination (i.e., pooping/peeing).

- **Exercise**
- **Non-Exercise Physical Activity** (NEPA). This is movement that isn't purposeful exercise, that still burns calories. For instance, gardening is not a deliberate attempt to improve strength or endurance, but it burns calories. Housework is not a deliberate attempt to improve your fitness, but it burns calories. Some people also just fidget. They sit there and bounce their ankle. Or they twirl their hair, or they click the pen. All these little things can add up to hundreds of calories per day.

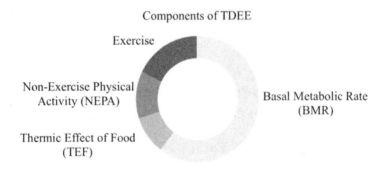

Components of TDEE

A drop in any one of these can cause weight gain. It also explains **why you might be eating the same number of calories as before, but still gaining weight**. The "calories in" part of the equation didn't change, but the calories out did.

Let's say that before menopause, your weight was stable, and hypothetically, you were eating 2500 calories a day. Since your weight was stable, you were also burning 2500 calories per day. Now that you've hit menopause, you're still eating 2500 calories per day, but you're now burning maybe 2300 calories per day. So what used to be maintenance calories is now a surplus of calories.

So **where did this drop in caloric expenditure come from**? Is it from metabolism or other sources? By and large, it's the other components of TDEE.

One very large study[70] looked at the metabolism of people as young as 8 days old, and as old as 95 years old. They found that strictly speaking about metabolism, **there is no difference between the age of 20 and 60**. Zero. Is weight gained during this time? For some people, yes, for others, no. But **if weight is gained, it's not due to a drop in metabolism. It's largely due to changes in activity levels and/or nutrition**. Maybe when you were 20, you would play pickup soccer a few times a week, and you're not doing that anymore when you're 60.

After 60, metabolism does slow down by up to 0.7% per year, which isn't a lot. So any weight gained beyond 0.7% per year is not due to metabolism slowing down.

One study[71] revealed that, during menopause, **weight gain primarily occurs due to a substantial decrease in NEPA** rather than a decline in BMR. So you're basically moving around less – involuntarily. You're less fidgety. In the words of the researchers, **"weight gain during menopause is predominantly due to a reduction in spontaneous activity**." These little things can add up to hundreds of calories per day.

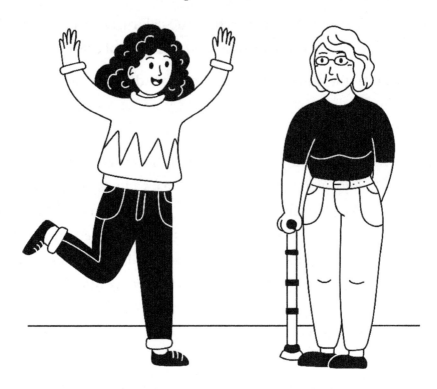

Fortunately, your metabolism doesn't slow down until approximately the age of 60, and even then, it slows down a little. But for the small declines in metabolism, what's the reason? The two biggest factors are simply body temperature, and muscle mass. As long as your body temperature is normal (36.5-36.8 Celsius or 97.7-98.2 Fahrenheit), there's not much to do there.

As for muscle mass – that's largely within your control. One study concluded that **the primary reason that metabolism slows down after menopause (and even then, not by much) is the loss of muscle**. Another study[72] found the same thing.

The solution to a decline in muscle mass is fairly simple (but not necessarily easy): **strength training and adequate protein**. Rea strength training. Not body pump classes. That's cardio with weights. Not that it's bad for you, but it's not strength training. How do you do strength training properly? Stay tuned until chapter 6, where we'll outline how to exercise properly during and after menopause. And in chapter 3, we'll discuss protein.

Myth #4: My Thyroid Caused the Weight Gain

We're often told that **the thyroid is the master metabolic gland**. Since it largely controls body temperature, it's largely responsible for the metabolic rate as well. So it's logical to conclude that since the metabolism slowed down (which we know is questionable, and the extent of the decrease is very small), the thyroid must be slowing down.

This one is only a half-myth, as you'll see. The story of what happens to thyroid with age is quite fascinating.

One systematic review[80] found that 2.4% of postmenopausal womenhave diagnosable thyroid disease. An additional 23.2% of postmenopausal women have subclinical thyroid disease (subclinical means that it's not bad enough to be a diagnosable disease, but not good enough to be considered normal). Within that group of 23.2% with subclinical thyroid disease, 73.8% is hypothyroid, and 26.2% is hyperthyroid.

Here's where it gets a bit tricky: **to diagnose thyroid issues, you have to use the right tests, and look at the right things**. The most used test for thyroid function is TSH (thyroid stimulating hormone). While it's a good test, it's not complete. Tests that give you additional information about thyroid function are:

- Total T4
- Free T4
- Total T3
- Free T3
- Reverse T3
- Thyroid binding globulin (TBG)
- Anti-TPO antibodies
- Anti-TGB antibodies

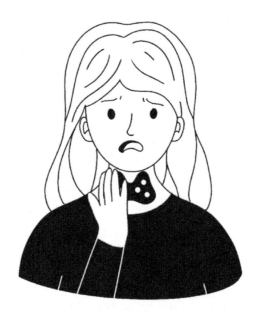

Although this isn't a book on thyroid physiology (though you can find a comprehensive video explaining these tests at www.Mastering-Menopause.com), the key takeaway is that relying solely on TSH doesn't provide a complete picture of thyroid function. Why? Because one study[5] showed that in postmenopausal women, **there aren't any changes in TSH, but there are drops in T4 and T3** (called "the active thyroid hormones"). In that study, the researchers recruited 50 healthy women between ages 20-44, and 50 healthy women between ages 45-77. Although both groups were healthy, the T4 levels of the older women were 37% lower than those of the younger women. The T3 levels of the older women were 16% lower than those of the younger women.

The real question from all of this is "what does that mean?" Should these drops in thyroid levels be addressed, or left alone?

One study[23] proposed that the slight decline in thyroid hormones might actually be a good thing. With a lower metabolic rate, you use less energy, which **contributes to longevity**.

But when do these declines in thyroid levels become excessive? When is it "Too much of a good thing?" If someone has had declines in their thyroid levels from before menopause to after menopause, and is not experiencing hypothyroid symptoms, chances are that no treatment may be necessary. But if their thyroid levels have dropped, and they are experiencing hypothyroid symptoms, it may be time to speak to their doctor about getting some treatment.

Or if all of this is too confusing, speak to your doctor anyway.

Myth #5: I'm Inflamed

Due to charlatan health gurus using scare tactics about inflammation, more and more people are afraid that they're inflamed. In fact, without testing, lots of people are claiming that they're inflamed. It's almost trendy to be inflamed. But **how does menopause affect inflammation**?

To really answer that, we have to look at the common tests for inflammation:

- CRP (C-Reactive Protein)
- TNF-alpha (Tumor Necrosis Factor alpha)
- IL-6 (Interleukin-6)
- Fibrinogen

By the way, if you want a list of the 49 blood tests that I give to my clients to ask their doctors to run, it's available to you for free at www.Mastering-Menopause.com.

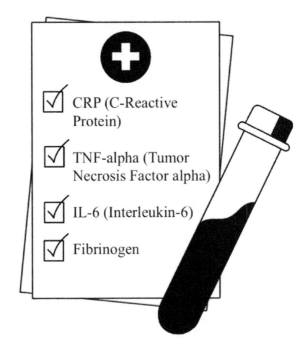

While this isn't a book on diagnostics, I just want to lay the groundwork for how inflammation is measured.

One study[85] compared the levels of CRP, IL-6 and TNF-alpha between 45 premenopausal women and 44 postmenopausal women. They found that CRP and IL-6 are no higher in the postmenopausal women compared to the premenopausal women, but TNF-alpha was indeed higher.

Another study[28] also found that fibrinogen is no different between premenopausal and postmenopausal women.

But let's backtrack a little bit, and ask a seemingly basic question: what is inflammation? The simple answer is that inflammation is a repair process. The body is trying to repair damaged tissue.

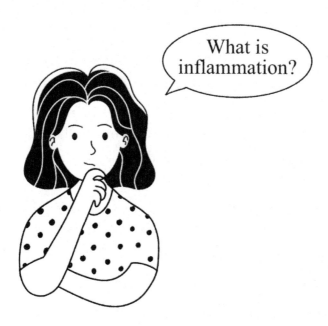

So what's damaged? What is the body trying to repair? Largely – it's the muscle that is lost with aging and declining estrogen levels. How do we know this? Because in one study[1], every inflammatory marker that was elevated decreased with both cardio and strength training. One large systematic review[50] of 1510 postmenopausal women found the same thing: **exercise is anti-inflammatory in postmenopausal women**.

Stay tuned until chapter 6 to learn how to exercise properly in your postmenopausal years.

Myth #6: I Should Gain Muscle to Lose Fat

This is another myth that spread during the early days of the internet. The myth went like this: "Muscle burns calories even when you're sleeping. So if you increase your muscle, you'll speed up your metabolism, and lose fat."

This is only partially true. The numbers thrown around on the internet until very recently were that each pound of muscle burns 40-50 calories per day. But anyone who actually did the math would see that it doesn't make sense. The body of an average postmenopausal woman (who doesn't do strength training) contains about 27% muscle. So if a woman weighs 150 pounds, she would have about 40 pounds of muscle. If each pound burned 40-50 calories per day, her metabolic rate from muscle alone would be 1600-2000 calories per day. Never mind all the calories burned by other organs (the brain and liver burn a lot of calories as well).

But metabolic rates for average postmenopausal women are around 900-1400 calories per day.

It is now estimated that **each pound of muscle burns around 6-10** calories per day. But that's not the whole story. **Body fat also burns calories**. It burns around 2 calories per pound per day.

So for the "gain muscle to burn fat" theory to be meaningful, you'd have to gain a lot of muscle. Like 15-20 pounds of muscle. And that's extremely difficult (and takes 2-3 years).

So gaining muscle to burn fat is not the most direct way to fat loss. There are many great reasons to gain muscle, like:

- Improved bone density.
- Better mobility, and overall function.
- Better blood sugar control.
- Lower blood pressure.
- Reduced inflammation.

But **fat loss is not a good reason to gain muscle**.

Myth #7: Fat Loss is 80% Nutrition and 20% Exercise

You'll often see this sound bite online – if you want to lose fat, nutrition is responsible for 80% of the results, and exercise is responsible for 20% of the results.

Unfortunately, sound bites lose a lot of nuances. And this sound bite is certainly not true for postmenopausal women.

At this stage of your life, **exercise is more like 40-50% of the fat loss puzzle.** Remember from myth #3, that **the biggest reason for fat gain during and after menopause is not a slowdown in metabolism, but a drop in involuntary activity**? Well, the way you compensate for that is with an **increase in voluntary activity** – exercise.

In one very large study[54], the researchers followed 34,079 women for 15 years. At the beginning of the study, their average age was 54 years old.

The women were divided into 3 categories based on their physical activity levels:

- Group 1 burned less than 7.5 calories/kg/week. In other words, a 154-pound woman is 70 kg. So this woman would have burned less than 525 calories per week.
- Group 2 burned between 7.5-21 calories/kg/week.
- Group 3 burned over 21 calories/kg/week.

To absolutely nobody's surprise, **the group that exercised the most gained the least weight** (between 0-2.3 kg or about 5 lbs.), while very few women lost weight. Again, this might be pointing to the fact that **the postmenopausal body actually wants to gain body fat to maintain whatever estrogen levels** can be maintained.

Myth #8: There's an Optimal Estrogen or Hormone Level

One common question amongst postmenopausal women is **"what's the optimal estrogen/progesterone/testosterone level?"**

We wish it were a nice, simple answer, like a specific number. But unfortunately, it's much more complicated than that. Here's why:

We use the word "estrogen" like it's a single hormone, but it's actually 3 different hormones:

- **Estradiol:** the dominant premenopausal estrogen. Largely made by the ovaries, although the adrenal glands and body fat make it as well.
- **Estrone:** the dominant postmenopausal estrogen. Largely made by body fat. And weaker than estradiol.
- **Estriol:** the dominant estrogen during pregnancy. Since that's not the topic of this book, we'll leave that one out of the conversation.

So one thing that makes it hard to determine an optimal hormone level is to determine which estrogen we're talking about.

Furthermore, **estrogen is a double-edged sword**. On the one hand, it improves bone density, mood, muscle, skin, decreases hot flashes, etc., but on the other hand, high levels of estrogen are also implicated in different cancers, like breast, vaginal, ovarian, endometrial, etc. So what's the right level that gives you the benefits of estrogen, without the risks of estrogen? We wish it was a strict cutoff, but it isn't. **There's some overlap.**

As if this wasn't complicated enough, the research is conflicting as well.

In one study, 209 postmenopausal women were given questionnaires about cognitive decline. The average estradiol levels in women <u>with</u> cognitive decline were 14.95 pg/ml (54.8 pmol/l). The average estradiol levels of women <u>without</u> cognitive decline were 21.67 pg/ml (79.6 pmol/l).

If you were to look at this single study, you'd conclude "A-ha! So the optimal level of estradiol after menopause is over 20 pg/ml (73.4 pmol/l)." But it's not quite that simple, because in the group that had

41

cognitive decline, their <u>average</u> estradiol level was 14.95 pg/ml (54.8 pmol/l). But the variation was ±10.24 pg/ml (37.6 pmol/l). It means that the range was as low as 4.71 pg/ml (17.3 pmol/l), and as high as 25.19 pg/ml (92.5 pmol/l). In the group that didn't have cognitive decline the <u>average</u> estradiol level was 21.67 pg/ml (79.6 pmol/l), but the range was ±14.92 pg/ml (54.8 pmol/l). So as you can see, there's significant overlap in estradiol levels between women who had cognitive decline and those who didn't.

Levels of Estradiol

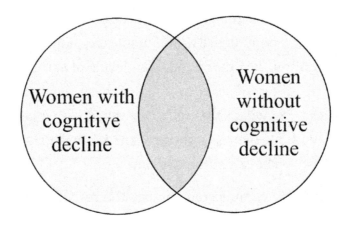

The same is true for other health outcomes, like heart health, osteoporosis, etc.

Case in point, in one study[26,] 90 postmenopausal women were recruited, and divided into 2 groups:

- Had a heart attack in the last year.
- Didn't have a heart attack in the last year.

The results are a bit confusing, because it's actually the group that didn't have a heart attack that had lower estrogen levels.

Here's the data:

	Heart Attack	No Heart Attack
Estrone	52 pg/ml (192.3 pmol/l)	29 pg/ml (107.3 pmol/l)
Estradiol	31 pg/ml (113.8 pmol/l)	13 pg/ml (47.7 pmol/l)

These are just two examples, but the literature is filled with conflicting and confusing data.

Because it's so complicated, women will often go to their endocrinologist, gynecologists, and GPs for years, trying different ratios of estradiol/estrone/progesterone every few months to figure out what's the right mix.

After all, if it was simple, we would just measure a woman's current hormone levels, and give her the amount of hormone that brought her up to ideal. But therein lies the problem: **we don't know what's ideal**, and likely, it varies woman-by-woman.

Myth #9: There's a Magic, Hormone-Balancing Superfood, Supplement or Device

Lots of superfoods, supplements or devices are marketed as "hormone-balancing." But there are 3 problems with that:

- You can see from the previous myth how complex "hormone balancing" really is.
- They don't specify which hormone(s) they balance.
- They have no evidence to back it up.

About the closest you can get to balancing all hormones is what I call the "**boring basics**": exercise 4+ days per week, good nutrition (adequate calories, adequate protein, adequate fibre), stress management and good sleep. Although for some women, making these lifestyle changes, sometimes isn't enough to adequately balance their hormones, and they need additional help.

Components of "boring basics"

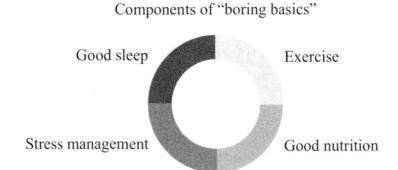

Good sleep

Exercise

Stress management

Good nutrition

Why is Weight Gained Around the Middle?

This one is not a myth, but more of an FAQ (frequently asked question), so I thought I'd put it in here.

Before menopause, most women tend to store their body fat in their buns and thighs. During and after menopause, the body fat shifts to the waist.

What caused this shift?

One of the things that regulates the location of your body fat is your hormones. A body fat distribution in the buns and thighs is **indicative of estrogen dominance** – which is what should be happening before menopause.

After menopause, **estrogen drops a lot, but testosterone only drops a bit.** So now, there's a **testosterone-to-estrogen ratio that favours testosterone more than before menopause.**

The other reason behind the shifting body fat towards the middle is an **increase in cortisol levels**[95,96]. Cortisol is also related to belly fat.

How do you get rid of belly fat? While **you can't spot reduce** (you can't reduce belly fat by doing abdominal exercises. They'll strengthen your abs, but won't make them any leaner), if you lose fat overall, you'll also lose belly fat. The other way to burn fat is through hormone balance and certain ratios of hormones/hormone profiles are related to certain fat distributions (for example, when a woman has more testosterone than estrogen, she'll have more belly fat than thigh fat. But when a woman has more estrogen than testosterone, she'll have more thigh fat than belly fat). However, if your primary fat storage place even before menopause was your belly, then it might just be genetics, and there's not much that can be done about it.

How Long do Menopausal Symptoms Last?

This is another FAQ that made sense to include in this chapter. One study[67] found large differences in the duration of menopausal symptoms. About 80% of women feel symptoms for 4 years and

10% of women feel symptoms for as much as 12 years. Why the variation? It largely depends on when a woman started experiencing hot flashes. If a woman started experiencing hot flashes before menopause, she'll have symptoms for an average of 11.8 years. But women who only started experiencing hot flashes after menopause will only feel symptoms for 3.4 years.

Of course, there are the cases of women who never experienced any symptoms whatsoever.

According to one study, ethnicity only changes the age of onset (some ethnicities experience an earlier menopause, and others a later menopause), but it appears that the duration of the menopausal symptoms is quite universal.

Chapter 3

The Menopause Diet

The 5 biggest concerns for postmenopausal women are:

- Body fat
- Menopausal symptoms
- Fracture risk/bone density
- Maintaining muscle strength (and function) into older age
- Heart health

Yes, there may be individual concerns, like diabetes, high blood pressure (which also kind of falls under heart health), and others, but the 5 almost universal concerns for menopausal women are the ones mentioned above.

In this chapter, you'll learn:

- How many calories should you eat if you want to lose weight?
- What foods to eat to reduce menopausal symptoms.
- An alcoholic beverage that's surprisingly good for menopausal symptoms (no, not red wine).
- How caffeine affects hot flashes.
- Menopause, bones and calcium – how much do you need?
- How to maintain lean muscle during and after menopause.
- Heart health: why it's more complicated than cholesterol and triglycerides.

If you do have specific concerns about type 2 diabetes and high blood pressure, I've written entire books on those topics, titled *Type 2 Diabetes Reversal Secrets* and *High Blood Pressure Reversal Secrets*. I've made the first chapter of these books available to you for free at www.Mastering-Menopause.com.

Without further ado, let's jump in.

How Many Calories Should You Eat?

The million-dollar question: how many calories should you eat? There are a million and one answers to this question, but my guess is that you're trying to lose fat. Why? Because someone trying to maintain their weight usually isn't asking this question. So, let's go with that assumption.

While there are a lot of calorie calculators out there, I like a very simple formula. Here's what it takes to <u>maintain</u> your weight:

Current bodyweight (in pounds) x 15 + calories spent on exercise.

Let's use an example. Let's say you weigh 150 pounds, and you don't currently exercise. So 150 x 15 = 2250. That's how many calories you currently eat in a day (knowingly or unknowingly). Let's say that you do exercise. You go for 60-minute walk 3 days a week. Each walk burns 200 calories. So you would divide 600 calories (3 walks per week x 200 calories per walk) by 7 (days per week). That comes to about 85 calories. This makes your current calories are 2250 + 85, or around 2335 calories.

Again, that's how many you're currently eating. If you want to lose body fat, typical advice would be to subtract 500 calories per day to lose 1 pound per week (because a pound of fat is 3500 calories). But here's the problem: **you want to reduce the "calories in" side of the equation, hoping that the "calories out" side of the equation is unchanged**. But frequently it does change.

Maybe you reduce your calories by 500 per day, but your body feels a little more lethargic, so you burn 200 fewer calories per day. You think you have a 500-calorie deficit, but it's really only a 300 calorie per day deficit. At the end of the week, you're not down a pound. You're down less than a pound. Or nothing. Or maybe, you're even up.

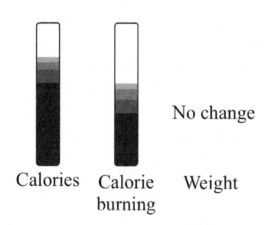

No change

Calories Calorie   Weight
          burning

The body fights back against caloric deficits that it perceives to be too large. So, my recommendation is to **start with a 10% deficit**. For instance, if you are eating 2500 calories per day, try cutting 250 calories per day. The key to long term fat loss is to cut calories that you won't miss. If you have a large caloric deficit, you'll get hungry... and go on a binge after a few days. Or sneak some food "when no one is looking."

Another problem with tracking calories is that I have yet to find an accurate app, software, etc. Their accuracy is atrocious, especially the big ones, like MyFitnessPal, Noom, MyPlate, LoseIt, etc.

One study[37] compared the accuracy of 5 different popular nutrition tracking apps with just a good ol' food diary and found that the nutrition tracking apps underestimated calories by as much as 27%.

Another study[89] found similar results.

And the vast majority of research that compares nutrition tracking apps basically finds the same thing: they are way way way off[10,16,45,64].

A lot of us lie to ourselves (and nutrition apps lie to us) about how much we're actually eating. We think we're eating 1800 calories per day, and we wonder why we aren't losing body fat. But the reality might be closer to 2700 (yep, with my clients I've seen estimates as far off as 40-50%).

Case in point, in one study[19], women who had a hard time losing body fat despite <u>thinking</u> they were eating a low number of calories were asked how many calories they ate per day. For the following 28 days, they were supplied with daily meals adding up to their self-reported calories. These women ended up losing about 1.7 pounds per week (0.75 kg) when they actually ate the number of calories that they thought they were eating.

Is that to say that a slow metabolism doesn't exist? No, slow metabolisms definitely exist. However, how wide is the gap between a person with a slow metabolism and a fast metabolism? According to this study[20], **less than 15%.**

To put some numbers to this, if a woman with a fast metabolism needs 2500 calories to maintain her weight, a woman with a slow metabolism (who has the same weight) needs around 2125 calories to maintain her weight.

So what gives? **Why the discrepancy between what people report (low calories) and what the research shows** (that when a caloric deficit exists, weight is lost)? There are a few possible reasons:

- **Food label reporting is off.** At least in North America, food labels are allowed to be off by as much as 20%. Twenty percent out of 2500 calories is 500. The food labels say you're eating 2500 calories per day, but the reality may be closer to 3000. So you don't have a 500-calorie deficit. You have maintenance calories.

- **Small calories sneak in there.** For instance, the label on a jar of peanut butter is for a flat tablespoon. But if you use a heaping tablespoon (and you lick off the peanut butter at the bottom of the spoon), you're getting 80-100% more calories than reported.

- Maybe someone has a good caloric deficit 5-6 days per week, and they have a **massive surplus over 1-2 days of the week** (like the weekends). This negates the deficit.

- Maybe they're **snacking mindlessly** They're eating while simultaneously doing something else (watching TV, working, etc.). Because they're not conscious of their eating, they underestimate how much they ate.

- Maybe you are losing body fat, but something is causing you to **retain water**, so fat weight is down, water weight is up, and the net effect (in the short term) is no weight loss. But if people had waited a few more weeks, their efforts would be reflected on the scale.
- As mentioned earlier, if you're using popular nutrition tracking apps, their accuracy is atrocious.

Unfortunately, as it stands right now, the best way to calculate calories, carbs, protein and fats is the old school way:

- Write down what you ate.
- Write down how much of it you ate.
- Look up the nutritional value in a nutrition database (either one that you look up or the one provided for you at www.Mastering-Menopause.com) and multiply the calories by the serving size.

In an ideal world, you'd **get body fat testing every 2 weeks** to see if your calorie calculations are on track. Why body fat testing, instead of just the scale? Because in a 2-week period, you might lose 1-2 pounds of fat, but if you had something salty to eat, you could gain 1-2 pounds of water. The scale would show no weight loss. But a body fat test would show a drop in body fat.

However, if you don't have access to body fat testing, don't weigh yourself more frequently than once every 2 weeks. If after a 2-week period, your weight is down (even half a pound), maintain your current deficit.

If after a 2-week period, your weight is the same or higher, and you're convinced that you've had a deficit, keep doing what you're doing and measure again in 2 more weeks. If after 4 weeks, your weight is still the same or higher, increase your deficit by another 10%.

If you're reading all of this and think "I picked up a menopause book – not a book that gives me math homework", don't worry. There's more than one way to create a caloric deficit. Some women like counting calories, and others don't. If you don't like counting calories, in the next chapter I have some great techniques for you that will help you reduce your calories without counting calories.

Foods That Reduce Menopausal Symptoms

A second common concern of menopausal women is the menopausal symptoms. Now we know how many calories we need to eat. But what should those calories consist of? If you're experiencing menopausal symptoms, at least some of your calories should be devoted to the foods in this section.

The most common menopausal symptom is hot flashes, but it's not the only symptom. There are others (that I probably don't need to tell you about), like mood swings, depression, fatigue, brain fog, urogenital changes (things like vaginal dryness, decreased libido, frequent urination, etc.), muscle and joint aches, etc.

Which foods help relieve those? That's what we'll cover in this section.

Flax Seeds

In one study[21], postmenopausal women were divided into 3 groups:

- Group 1: took 500 mg of flaxseed extract (a capsule).
- Group 2: ate 2 tablespoons of flax seeds per day.
- Group 3: took a collagen supplement.

At the end of 6 months, the results were:

Group	Overall Menopausal Symptoms	Hot Flash Intensity
Flaxseed extract	Reduced by 25%	Reduced by 26%
Flax seeds (2 tablespoons)	Reduced by 30%	Reduced by 23%
Placebo	Reduced by 11%	Reduced by 3%

Conclusion: **flaxseeds help reduce overall menopausal symptoms**, as well as hot flashes.

What was the mechanism? It's been theorized that flaxseeds exert their action through a mild estrogenic effect, but this study disproved that, because the **levels of estradiol were unchanged over the 6-month duration**. The researchers did not venture a guess as to why flaxseeds (both dietary and supplemental) improved menopausal symptoms. One thing I personally would have liked to have seen is a measurement of estrone. As we know from the previous chapter, it's **estrone that's the dominant postmenopausal estrogen**, but unfortunately in this study, they didn't measure it.

Regardless of the reason, the result is clear: flax seeds (both as a food and as a supplement) reduce menopausal symptoms.

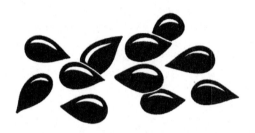

A larger meta-analysis[31] found the same thing.

Soy and Tofu

Soy and tofu are a frequent staple and recommendation for postmenopausal women. They have a **mild estrogenic effect**, so it's theorized that as a result, they help reduce menopausal symptoms. One study[8] put the theory to the test.

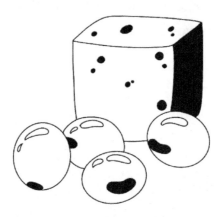

In this study, researchers recruited 75 women, between ages 45-50 who had their last period more than 1 year earlier.

After 3 months of daily soy consumption, they had mild reductions (3-8%) in the following symptoms:

- Hot flashes
- Sweating
- Excessive bleeding
- Sleeping problems
- Depression
- Irritability
- Vaginal dryness
- Anxiety
- Joint and muscle discomfort

Another study[27] recruited 25 perimenopausal women and had them consume tofu daily for 3 months. There was a similar finding to the previous study – reductions in menopausal symptoms (specifically, hot flashes, incontinence, painful intercourse, frequent urination, and insomnia).

Most of the research does indeed find a benefit of soy and tofu on menopausal symptoms.

I know some readers of this book will ask "Maybe it's good for menopausal symptoms, but doesn't it raise the cancer risk?"

While that's a discussion for a whole other book (and several have been written), the short answer is that on a population basis, **soy actually lowers cancer risk**. In one meta-analysis[92], there was an inverse relationship between tofu consumption and breast cancer risk. Another meta-analysis[66] found the same thing. That's on a population basis. On an individual basis, the answer might be different, so if you want the answer as it pertains to you, seek the help of a registered dietitian who specializes in cancer.

Beer

This is the section that might be worth the price of this book alone. Did you know that beer can have a positive impact on menopausal symptoms, without having a negative effect on your health otherwise? It's true!

In one study[90], 37 postmenopausal women were divided into 3 groups:

- Alcoholic beer (330 ml/day)
- Non-alcoholic beer (660 ml/day)
- Control

After 6 months, the results were surprising:

Compared to the control group, here's what happened:

Symptoms	Alcoholic Beer	Non-Alcoholic Beer
Somatic	Decreased by 22%	Decreased by 20%
Psychological	Decreased by 42%	Decreased by 22%
Urogenital	Decreased by 8%	Decreased by 2%

If you're wondering about what the different symptoms mean, here are examples:

- **Somatic symptoms**: headaches, joint pain, muscle pain.
- **Psychological symptoms**: anxiety, difficulty concentrating (brain fog), forgetfulness.
- **Urogenital symptoms**: vaginal dryness, decreased libido, frequent urination.

The message: drink beer! But if you're following the advice from the previous section (about calories), work it into your "caloric budget." In other words, if you're "allowed" 2500 calories per day, and you do want to drink beer, subtract the beer calories from your total calories.

And this isn't an isolated study to prove my personal biases (not that it matters, but my personal bias is I don't like beer. I actually don't drink any alcohol. Bubble tea is my vice). Another study[3] found similar results: **beer improves menopausal symptoms**.

If you're a beer lover, you're probably so giddy right now, you don't care about the mechanism, but for the curious reader, I'll explain. Beer is made of hops, and hops are estrogenic (for the geeks, the estrogenic part is called "isoxanthohumol").

You're welcome for that justification to drink beer. Although gluten-free beer wasn't studied for its effect on menopausal symptoms, my opinion is that yes, it would also decrease them. Gluten is a protein, and the estrogenic part of beer is hops/isoxanthohumol. I don't believe that part is affected by the removal of gluten.

Caffeine and Hot Flashes

You might have seen this section title and gotten nervous. "You're giving me beer in one section, but taking away my coffee?" Fear not.

One study[29] compared one group of women complaining of hot flashes to another group of women who didn't. The researchers tried to see if there are any differences in coffee consumption between the 2 groups. Fortunately, there was a negligible difference between the 2 groups, and no differences in other menopausal symptoms (sleep, bowel, bladder, and sexual function).

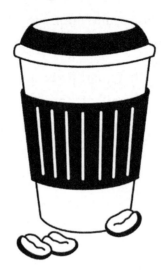

So enjoy your cuppa Joe.

Menopause, Bones and Calcium

One of the greatest concerns of postmenopausal women is **breaking a bone**. So they pay extra attention to calcium. They eat more dairy, take more calcium supplements, all in an effort to reduce fracture risk.

While I agree that it's extremely important to prevent fractures, unfortunately research shows[48] that calcium (both in food and supplements) is not the way to do that. Surprising, I know.

I wrote a book on this that goes into full detail, called *Osteoporosis Reversal Secrets*. The first chapter is available to you for free at www.Mastering-Menopause.com.

So if calcium is not what helps reduce fracture risk, what does? Protein!

How to Maintain Lean Muscle During and After Menopause

Fortunately, protein accomplishes more than one goal – **it's good not just for your muscles, but your bones as well.**

Lots of women are concerned about their fracture risk, and declining strength and function, as their estrogen declines. The fear is either needing to be dependent on caregivers or loved ones or having to live in a home.

While the jury is still out on how much protein is optimal, here are a few clues:

One study[55] found that postmenopausal women with a protein consumption of 1.2 g/kg/day had greater strength than women with a lower protein intake, even though muscle mass was the same.

In one study[36], women aged 60-90 had better physical performance, muscle mass, and lower fat when their protein intake was higher (1.1 g/kg/day), compared with women who had intakes of under 0.8 g/kg/day.

Though in my opinion, even the high amounts of protein used in these studies is still low. Protein requirements depend on 3 major factors:

- Your activity levels.
- Your weight.
- Your age.

Here's how it breaks down:

Activity Level	Under 60	Over 60
Sedentary	0.8-1.2 grams/kg/day	1.2-1.8 grams/kg/day
Cardio only	1.2-1.4 grams/kg/day	1.8-2.1 grams/kg/day
Strength training only	1.6-1.8 grams/kg/day	2.4-2.7 grams/kg/day
Cardio + strength training	1.6-1.8 grams/kg/day	2.4-2.7 grams/kg/day

You might notice that the **protein requirements of people over 60 are higher than those under 60**. Why is that? Because folks over 60 have worse absorption than those under 60, so their protein requirements are quite a bit higher according to one systematic review[6].

If you don't feel like doing math, and you just want to plug your details into a calculator, so it'll just tell you how much protein you should be getting, enter your email at www.Mastering-Menopause.com, and you'll get a link to the protein calculator.

Now that you know how much you need, let's talk about the best protein sources. Simply put, **the best protein sources are meat, fish and seafood** (plus a couple of modified foods, which you'll see in a second), not dairy, eggs (but as you'll see in a second, egg whites are also a great protein source), beans, lentils, nuts or tofu.

Here is a list of what I call "Grade A" protein. What makes the following foods Grade A? Each of them has **over 30 grams of protein per serving**.

- Chicken
- Turkey
- Beef
- Veal
- Pork
- Lamb
- Duck
- Shrimp
- Crab
- Lobster
- Calamari
- Tuna
- Cod
- Tilapia
- Salmon
- Sardines
- Low fat dairy (like skim milk, low fat/no fat yogurt, cottage cheese, etc.)
- Protein powders
- Egg whites

Next is a list of what I would call "Grade B" protein. What makes these Grade B? They have between 10 25 grams of protein per serving.

- Beans

- Lentils
- Greek yogurt
- Tofu
- Protein bars
- Quinoa
- Chickpeas
- Peanut butter
- Hemp seeds
- Oats/oatmeal

By the way, these lists of Grade A and Grade B protein aren't exhaustive. There are other foods in those categories, but I can't include every single food in existence in this book. If you're wondering about a specific food that's not listed here, visit www.Mastering-Menopause.com, and I'll send you a website where you can look up the protein content of different foods.

For the sake of completeness, I'm going to add in a third section: foods people say are good sources of protein, but really aren't... plus the reasons people say they're a good source of protein.

Nuts: unlike chicken for instance, where 150-200 grams is a pretty normal serving, most people wouldn't have 150-200 grams of nuts. Most people might have a handful of nuts, which is around 30 grams. Most nuts have a very similar nutrition profile, whether it's almonds, cashews, pecans, walnuts, pistachios, etc. In general, 30 grams of nuts have about 6-7 grams of protein. Not much. But if you were to have even 150 grams of nuts (they're all pretty similar in calories), you certainly get 30-35 grams of protein... but along with that, you'd also get 66 grams of fat, 124 grams of carbs, and a whopping 800+ calories. By comparison, 150-200 grams of grilled chicken (for instance) would give you about 45-60 grams of protein, 0 carbs, and only 5-7 grams of fat. For a total of around 300 calories.

Eggs: a medium egg has about 6 grams of protein. On its own, it's not a great protein source. But if you have 2 or more eggs together, it amounts to something. Again, this does not apply to egg whites. Egg whites are considered a "Grade A protein."

Peas: a cup of peas only has about 8 grams of protein.

Milk: a cup of milk has 9 grams of protein.

Cheese: if you had cheese in the same quantity you have meat (150-200 grams or more), it would be a Grade B protein. But you don't. A serving size for cheese is usually a slice or a cube. A slice of cheese is about 30 grams, so that's 1 serving. Most cheeses (cheddar, havarti, mozzarella, gouda, etc.) are similar in their protein content. One slice of cheese has 8-9 grams of protein. So if you were to have 2+ slices, it would be considered Grade B protein.

Yogurt: a cup of yogurt has about 5-6 grams of protein. Greek yogurt is higher, which is why it's Grade B.

Chia seeds: like many of these other foods, you wouldn't eat chia seeds in the same quantities you'd eat meat. You'd typically have chia seeds somewhere between a teaspoon and a tablespoon. A tablespoon of chia seeds contains only about 2 grams of protein.

If you're wondering "*But Igor, what about food X?*" that I didn't list here, fear not. I'll provide you a link where you can check the protein content of different foods if you just visit www.Mastering-Menopause.com.

Heart Health

When it comes to nutrition for heart health, let's just say, **it's complicated**. To evaluate how any given food affects heart health, we'd need to have 2 groups of women eating the same diet for a lifetime, with only one difference: maybe one group of women eats vegetables, and another doesn't (everything else is the same – calories, exercise, smoking, etc.). At the end of their lives, the causes of death are analyzed, and a firm conclusion can be made.

Because such research doesn't exist (and probably never will), **"proxy markers"** need to be used. These are markers that are believed to have some kind of relationship to heart health. We need this to make the conclusion that if a certain food or diet changes a proxy marker, it also changes the risk of heart disease.

Examples of proxy markers are things like cholesterol, triglycerides, inflammation, and others.

Whether any of these markers have a relationship to heart disease is still complicated, confusing, and nuanced. For instance, after we learned of the existence of cholesterol, we then learned that there are 2 types of cholesterol: HDL and LDL. The lay public started calling them "good" cholesterol (HDL) and "bad" cholesterol (LDL). While that's a gross oversimplification, let's ask an important question: if LDL cholesterol is indeed the bad cholesterol, does it have any relationship to heart disease? That part isn't clear.

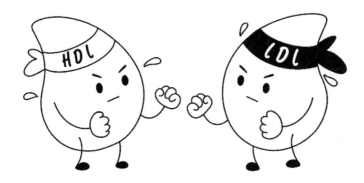

In one study[4] of 485 people, there appeared to be no relationship between levels of total cholesterol, LDL cholesterol, HDL cholesterol and triglycerides and death. So regardless of whether a person's levels were high or low, it didn't predict their risk of dying. Yet, in a different meta-analysis[56], there was an association between levels and death.

Confused? Wait until the end of this chapter, and I'll give you my 2 cents.

So **the relationship between cholesterol and heart disease is complicated, confusing, and far from conclusive**.

Because of that, scientists started to look for other blood markers that could be predictive of heart disease.

Inflammation was a good theory, so scientists started looking into the links between inflammation and heart disease. One **inflammatory marker often studied is CRP** (C-Reactive Protein), and its related test, hsCRP (high sensitivity C-Reactive Protein).

The investigation began – **do elevated levels of CRP predict heart disease**? That's what one study[98] of 10,388 people attempted to answer. And the answer is unfortunately more complicated than a simple "yes" or "no." Here's what they found:

- People with a CRP level of >3 mg/L had a 110% higher risk of dying compared to people with a level <1 mg/L. This is if their CRP levels were high due to lifestyle.
- But if their CRP levels were high due to genetics, there was no relationship between CRP levels and mortality.
- In east Asians, lower CRP levels are predictive of death. In this population, a CRP level of over 1.2 increased the risk of death by 41-95%. In non-east Asians, a CRP level of 1.2 presents a pretty low risk of death.
- **CRP is a consequence of hidden inflammation** – not a cause of it.

What about other blood markers? What else might have a relationship with heart attacks and strokes?

Another one that's been proposed is **iron**. One well-established measurement of iron is **serum ferritin,** which has been proposed to have an effect on heart disease. But just like cholesterol, some studies show an association between ferritin levels and heart disease, and others don't.

Because there's still so much that we don't know about what blood markers have great predictive value in terms of heart disease, the optimal diet for postmenopausal women is still up in the air.

However, if I were to give strictly my opinion on heart health, I'd venture to say that likely, the two most important factors are extremely simple:

- Eat the right number of calories.
- Make sure most of those calories are single-ingredient foods. For instance, how many ingredients are in a tomato? Just 1: tomato. How many ingredients are in chicken? Just 1: chicken. How many ingredients are in ice cream? More than 1.

Are other things important as well? Probably, but likely a lot less than these 2 factors. Case in point – there are some cultures whose diets are predominantly meat, and others that are predominantly veggies – and both have equally good heart health. There are cultures that are extremely high in carbs (the ones living around the equator), and others extremely high in fat (like Inuit) – and both have equally good heart health.

For all the dietary differences between many cultures around the world, the commonalities are that they eat the right number of calories, and only single-ingredient foods.

Not to mention that the other factors make a big difference to heart health as well, like exercise (which we'll cover in chapter 6), stress management, and sleep (which we'll cover in chapter 9).

Chapter 4

End Emotional Eating

If we're older than the age of 5, chances are we already know what to eat – **more protein, more veggies, less junk**. Then why can't we stick to it? Because as I always say in my presentations, and to my readers, "**Information isn't motivation**." Just knowing good information is not enough for long-term behaviour change.

The real reasons people can't or don't eat what they know they should, are:

- Emotional eating,
- Stress eating,
- Lack of planning, and
- Cravings.

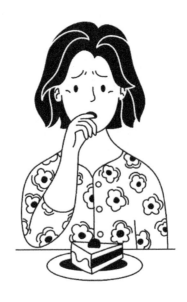

Think about these scenarios: you know you *should* have a chicken salad. But you just want some chocolate. You know you *should* have oatmeal with berries for breakfast, but you don't have any oatmeal or berries in the fridge. You brought a salad to work with you for lunch, but it's a colleague's birthday party, so there's cake and pizza. You know you *should* eat the salad you brought for lunch, but pizza and cake just taste so much better.

Do any of these scenarios seem familiar?

Would a diet/meal plan solve these problems? No. Because **the problem isn't nutritional**. That's only a surface level problem. **The real problems are emotional, logistical, and behavioural**. And we don't solve those kinds of problems with nutritional solutions. In this chapter, my goal is to at least get you started on the path to long-term nutritional behaviour change, without another diet or meal plan.

So let's dive in and explore different strategies that help you **cut calories without missing those calories**.

The following are strategies that my team and I actually use with our clients to get them to lose weight without putting them on another diet.

In no particular order:

Rate Your Hunger and Fullness

We often eat without being hungry. Maybe there's food around. Maybe it's "just time" to eat. But we don't really ask ourselves whether we're even hungry. Let's change that.

Next time, right before you sit down to eat, **rate your hunger and fullness on a -10 to +10 scale**. Between -10 and -1 means you're hungry (-10 means you're so hungry that your belly button is sticking to your spine and -1 means you're feeling mildly peckish). Between +1 and +10 means you're full (+10 means you're so full, you could swear you're 9 months pregnant with triplets and +1 means you're just slightly full).

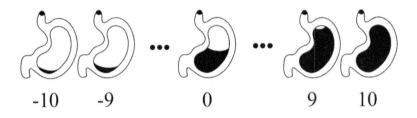

What does this do for you? If before a meal, you rate yourself as +2, it means that you're not hungry. Then you have to consciously or subconsciously justify to yourself why you're eating. Because **if your score is above a 0, you're eating for reasons other than hunger**.

My recommendation is **if you're thinking about eating, and you rate yourself more than 0, keep waiting**. Push back your mealtime. **Wait until you're hungry to eat**.

This is a very concrete exercise to help you "listen to your body." Because **there's only 1 good reason to eat: "I'm hungry."** There are also a million bad reasons to eat, like:

- I'm upset.
- I'm tired.
- I'm unfocused.
- It's time to eat.

- I'm excited.
- There's food around.

...etc.

If you've been eating for reasons other than hunger for years or decades, you might find this exercise challenging. It might even take you weeks or months to wait for hunger to eat, but the results will be well worth it.

Case in point – one of my clients, a 59-year-old woman, gained about 20 pounds since menopause and wanted to lose it. This was the strategy that I gave her. Nothing else. I didn't tell her to eat more veggies, or less junk, or give any other advice. I just told her to use this strategy. And over a period of about 6 months, she lost 20 pounds – without restriction.

Name the Emotion

If we lead busy lives, we sit down to eat even though we're feeling something else. Maybe we're excited, sad, tired, unfocused, anxious, surprised, or a myriad of other emotions. So next time before you eat, **name the emotion that you're feeling**.

The goal (as the title of this chapter suggests) is to end emotional eating. The first step to end emotional eating is to **create awareness of which emotions we're feeling**.

This is a simple, short exercise, but don't confuse its simplicity with a lack of effectiveness. It's actually quite effective. In essence, what you're doing is **creating psychological contrast between hunger and emotion**.

Mindful Eating

Mindful eating has become a real cliché over the last several years. It has taken on an almost pseudo-spiritual meaning.

But at its essence, mindful eating is extremely simple. **When you're eating – just eat**. Don't do anything else. Don't watch TV, don't scroll through your phone, don't work, don't read the newspaper.

Why is this important? A couple of reasons:

- If you're eating and simultaneously doing something else, you're **paying less attention to your fullness signals**, so you may end up eating beyond necessity.
- You want your **mealtimes to be distinct events in your memory**. If you're eating while doing something else, you may be storing that memory as "working" – but to your waist, it's still eating. So you end up not recalling what and how much you had earlier in the day, or the previous day.

Sounds logical, and this alone may be one of the most powerful things you can do to address mindless eating.

Rapid-Fire Ideas to Address Emotional Eating and Mindless Snacking

Besides the strategies covered earlier, here are some additional ideas to address emotional eating and mindless snacking:

- Feel like chewing something? **Chew gum**. It satisfies the craving to chew, but you get minimal to no calories.

- Want another way to get something in your mouth, without calories (get your mind out of the gutter)? **Drink water or tea**. Often, hunger is confused for thirst. So if you think you're hungry, try drinking water or tea, and wait for 15 minutes. If after 15 minutes, you're still hungry, it's probably real hunger. If after 15 minutes you forgot that you wanted to eat, great!
- Is it time to eat, but you're not feeling hungry? **Go for a walk**. Even if it's just 2-5 minutes. It may help you deal with the emotions without eating.
- Eating because you need a distraction? Try either **scrolling through social media** or **calling a friend/family member** to chat.

Pre-Plan Your Meals

One of the reasons we eat emotionally is because we don't think ahead of time about what we're going to eat. So when it comes to a mealtime, we're hungry. Or if we're not hungry, we're going to eat anyway, because it's "time to eat." Unless we've thought about what we're going to eat ahead of time, we'll pick the tastiest and most convenient thing. Unfortunately **the tastiest and most convenient thing is rarely the healthiest thing**.

That's where pre-planning comes in. What you need to do is very simple: when you wake up in the morning, **take 30 seconds to write down what you plan to eat that day**. It doesn't have to be super healthy. **It just has to be planned**. Want a pizza? Write it down. Want a chocolate cake? Write it down.

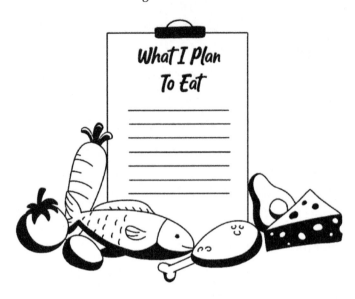

The real power in writing down your plan is **it doesn't feel like a cheat meal**. Imagine this (probably very familiar) scenario: you go on a diet. By day 5, you cheat on the diet. So you blow the diet and decide to restart after weeks or months.

However, if you planned to have chocolate cake, and you indeed had the chocolate cake, then you just followed the plan. It's not a slip-up. **It's part of the plan**. You didn't blow your diet. You followed the plan.

I want to emphasize not to overlook this strategy/technique just because it takes 30 seconds.

As mentioned earlier, **long-term behaviour change only happens when change is both easy and tasty**. Thirty seconds is easy.

It also addresses the obstacle of mindless snacking. **Mindless snacking happens when you haven't pre-planned your meals and snacks**. But if you've done the thinking earlier in the day, you don't have to do the thinking later in the day. If snacking wasn't part of the plan to begin with, you're less likely to mindlessly snack. If the snack was planned, chances are it'll be a mindful snack (and hopefully a healthy one, too).

Environmental Design for Healthy Eating

When Google was first starting out, they wanted to treat their employees really well. Part of that was never going hungry. So snacks were available anywhere within a matter of just a few steps. What did they have for snacks? Really delicious things, like:

- Chips
- Cookies
- Popcorn
- Pop
- Milkshakes

Their employees loved it. But **their waistlines didn't**. Neither did their doctor, once they started showing up for their yearly blood tests with elevated cholesterol, triglycerides, blood sugar, blood pressure, and others.

So what did Google do to turn that around?

You can't just take away something that everyone likes. Once you've had something, you can't get rid of it.

So, they didn't get rid of it, but instead, they made it **harder to access**. Instead of just taking a few steps and grabbing these snacks, they were now in cupboards. So you had to walk farther, and you couldn't just turn your head, and see delicious snacks in plain sight. If each time you turn your head, you see a snack, **you'll eat just because something is available**. Not because you're hungry. But if there's nothing in plain sight, constantly reminding and tempting you, it's much easier to not eat/drink it.

It didn't end there.

Not only did Google want to **discourage unhealthy snacking, but they also wanted to encourage healthy snacking**. So, what did they do?

They brought in additional snacks: **vegetables**. And the vegetables were put in plain sight, and closer than the cupboards where the unhealthy snacks were. So, there was a **constant reminder that vegetables were nearby**, and you had to exert less effort to get them than the other snacks.

As for the drinks, now they **featured water in beautiful water coolers, and made it look very presentable, with ice, and bits of oranges and lemons** floating in there. It just looked so refreshing.

Like with the vegetables, the water was now in plain sight and close, whereas the pop and milkshakes were out of plain sight and farther.

What happened to the waistlines and health markers of Google employees? Everything improved. Their **waistlines shrunk, their cholesterol, triglycerides, blood sugar and blood pressure all decreased**.

You can use the same principles to help yourself avoid foods that aren't conducive to good health.

The simplest (but not always easiest) way is to just **keep it out of the house**. After all, out of sight, out of mind. You want to make it so that if you want **the foods that are your vices, you have to exert more effort to get them**. You have to leave your house, walk/drive to where they sell your desired food, buy it, and bring it back home. What a hassle.

Sometimes though, that's not practical. Maybe you don't live by yourself. Maybe you like some foods that aren't conducive to your health, but someone in your household likes them as well. It wouldn't be nice if you took it away from other people. In those cases, you can try doing what Google did: either get them out of plain sight or **have the other people you live with hide your vice food, and not tell you where it is**.

I'm a chocoholic. I LOOOOOOVVVVVEEEE chocolate. Moderation goes out the window when chocolate is around me. I'll eat it even when I'm not hungry. But my wife is different. She can be satisfied with just one. On the rare occasion that I do have chocolate in my home, I ask my wife to hide it, and not tell me where it is. And that's good enough for me. I know it's at home, but the effort and time that I would have to exert to find that chocolate is not worth it to me. So it's not even tempting.

For one of my clients, her vice was Nutella, but it was her son buying it all the time. I told her the strategy of getting her son to hide it, but she was too good at finding it. So that wasn't an option. If we couldn't make it inaccessible, we had to pull another lever. We had to figure out **how to make Nutella undesirable**. I asked her what foods she hated. Right away, rosemary came to mind.

I recommended that every time she found Nutella at home, she put rosemary in it. That made Nutella less desirable to her. So she stopped eating it. As a nice side effect, her son was angry enough at this, that he just stopped buying it as well.

Reward Yourself

To reinforce good behaviour, you have to reward yourself. No, not with food. That's what we're trying to get away from. There are 4 criteria for a good reward:

- Free.
- Takes less than 1 minute.
- Has to feel good.
- You can do immediately after the desired behaviour.

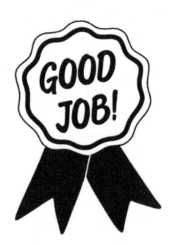

The reason that the reward has to be immediate is so that you can have a positive association with the behaviour.

There's a **difference between rewards and incentives**. **Rewards are immediate and happen every time after a desired behaviour**. Incentives are delayed (by weeks/months usually), and only happen when reaching milestones.

There's a time and a place for both, but an effective reward has to meet these 4 criteria. What are some examples of good rewards?

- Self-massage.
- Tell yourself you did a good job.
- Crack your knuckles or some other joint if you find it enjoyable, etc.

These are just examples. Use these or come up with ones that work for you.

Analyze and Adapt

What will likely happen is you'll pick a technique that appeals to you. Things will be going well at first, until you slip. The key is **doing a post-mortem**. Analyze why you slipped and figure out ways to avoid that in the future.

Most diets fail for the simple reason that we think it'll be no problem doing them. But there's a discrepancy between our plan and real-life. We plan for the best-case scenario. But **real life is not a best-case scenario**.

One of the keys to long-term behaviour change is planning for the worst-case scenario, not the best-case scenario. You have to **anticipate the obstacles that you might encounter along the**

way. Otherwise, they catch you by surprise. But if you've already anticipated them in your mind, you might have even come up with a way around them before they happen.

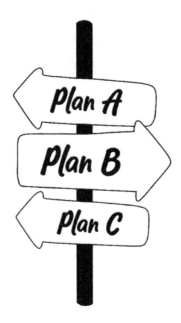

You now have one of the simplest, and yet, most powerful methods for behaviour change. The way I recommend you approach is to simply **pick a single strategy** from this chapter, and that's it. Master that one strategy. Stick with it, until you've been consistent with it for at least 3 months. After that, evaluate if you need additional strategies. You may or you may not. Case in point, as you'll learn in chapter 11, about Stellis – she just used 2 crazy simple strategies to lose 6 inches off her waist and get to her ideal weight. She didn't need everything. But she mastered one, until she needed another. **We're looking for simplicity. Not complexity**.

Chapter 5

How to Build Healthy Habits

You know you *should* exercise. You know you *should* eat better. And roughly speaking, you probably already know what to eat – more veggies, more protein, less junk. Pretty much every diet agrees on that.

So why don't you do it?

Because, as I often say in my presentations, **information isn't motivation**. Just knowing what to do isn't enough.

So **how do you establish the healthy habits that you know you _should_ have?**

That's what we'll discuss in this chapter.

The Battle Between the Emotional and Logical

In their book, *Switch: How to Change Things When Change is Hard*[41], psychologists Chip and Dan Heath say that the emotional side of the brain is like an elephant, and the logical side of the brain is like the person riding the elephant. So logically, you might know what you need to do (strength training, for example), but your emotions/feelings are pulling you in another direction (stay on the couch, watch Netflix, and snack on some chips or cookies). Sure, the rider gives direction, but the elephant is much stronger, so if there's a battle between the emotional and the logical side of the brain, the emotional will <u>always</u> win.

The key is to **align your emotions with your logic**. How do you do that? You ask yourself (or better yet, get someone else to ask) provocative questions that evoke emotion.

Questions That Evoke Emotion

You know logically that you need to exercise and eat healthier. Now how do you create an emotional connection to that? By digging deep with good questions.

So here are the questions that you ask to motivate yourself:

1. Why do I want to _____ (exercise/eat right)?

Keep asking "why" 3-5 times.

Example:

Q: Why do I want to exercise?

A: So that I can look good and have more energy.

Q: Why do I want to look good and have more energy?

A: Because I feel like I could get more done in my day if I had more energy.

Q: Why?

A: Because right now, there are lots of things I want to do that aren't getting done, because I just feel too tired.

And so on...

2. How do I expect to feel as a result of _____ (your goal)?

Don't just answer "Good" or "Happy." Elaborate on that.

3. If I keep doing what I am doing right now, what will happen in 6 months?

Paint yourself a **vivid picture**. The answer might be "I'll be even weaker, with even less energy. I'll avoid doing activities that I like to do, because I'm not happy with the way I look in my favourite clothes. I'll be less social. I won't go out with my partner or friends as much."

4. If I change what I'm doing now, and get on the right track, what will be the outcome in 6 months?

Again, don't just answer "That would be good" or "I will be happy." Instead, make it precise, vivid and detailed. Maybe the answer would be "If I were leaner, I'd get back into the clothes that I like to wear, go out more with my friends or husband, get more work done in my day, and have energy left over."

And of course, based on your answer, there may or may not be follow-up questions. That's why I recommend having someone else ask you these questions, so that as an objective person, they can think of intelligent follow-ups. Best to get someone experienced to ask these.

These questions are obviously very deep and require some soul-searching. If you do want to do these on your own, I recommend doing it in a distraction-free environment. Write them out on a piece of paper and answer them by hand. Not on your computer, because there are too many distractions on your computer (other windows/tabs, etc.). Carve out enough time (that might be 30-60 minutes), so that you give this exercise its proper time and attention, because the implications for your long-term success are huge.

Redefine "Success": Focus on Behaviors, Not Outcomes

You can't control your weight. You can influence it, but you can't control it. However, what you can control is whether you exercise and eat well. After all, if you exercise and eat right, but the weight isn't moving, then if the focus is the outcome (weight), you'll be disappointed. But if your focus is on the behavior (I will strength train 3 times in the next week), you'll feel a sense of accomplishment once you complete it.

So, you basically change the definition of success from something you can't control (your weight) to something that you can control (the number of times per week that you exercise).

And small accomplishments build on each other. You start to crave that feeling of accomplishment, so your consistency improves over time. But again, focus on what you can control.

Make Small Changes

The more things you try to change at the same time, the less likely you are to stick with them. For example, if you go on a high protein diet and it's drastically different from the way you currently eat, when you eat around your friends and family, there's going to be a strong "pull" to revert to your previous ways.

But if you make one tiny change, it won't be a big impediment. And after 2-12 weeks, when the change you've made feels really easy, natural and a regular part of your lifestyle, pick one more tiny little change and implement that. Continue repeating with newer habits. This way, if you implement one small habit per month, after a year you'll have a drastically healthier lifestyle, without really putting much effort into it.

The mentality I often recommend when it comes to healthy eating and exercise is to look at it as "**skill practice**."

For instance, if you've ever played an instrument, you know that it takes more than just a single class to become a maestro. If you've ever played a sport, you know that it takes more than just a single practice session to become good at it. The way you approach either of those is that you focus on just one tiny little skill for a few classes/sessions, until you become really good at that little skill. After that, you pick the next skill that builds on the one you just got good at, and so on.

That's the process of going from beginner to advanced.

If you were to apply the same mentality and process to healthy eating and exercising, you'd be much more successful at it than if you think of it as a "diet."

The **key, however, is to truly make the habit so easy that even you think it's ridiculous**. When you ask yourself "On a 0-10 scale, how confident am I that I can do _____ (fill in the blank with "exercise for 10 minutes per day" or "have 2 salads per week", or whatever else you like)?", the answer should be "9" or "10." It should be a no-brainer.

If your answer is "Maybe" or "I'll try", make your chosen behavior even easier.

Imagine these two contrasting scenarios:

You want to lose body fat, so you go on the internet, and read about the best diet for menopause. You see people losing fat, having more energy, and getting more toned. You want to try it too. But it's drastically different than your current diet.

Here's your current diet:

- Breakfast: coffee and a muffin.
- Lunch: turkey sandwich.
- Dinner: bowl of pasta in alfredo sauce, and for dessert, a couple of cookies. Along with that, you have a couple of glasses of wine.

Here's your new diet, that's amazing for weight loss:

- Breakfast: veggie omelet with a glass of water.
- Lunch: chicken, broccoli and rice.
- Dinner: baked asparagus and salmon.

How different is the new diet than the old diet? Drastically. It might be healthier, but it's going to be really difficult to stick to.

Compare that to using the "skill practice" method of healthy eating. Rather than doing a complete overhaul to your diet, maybe you just want to practice the "skill" of eating a better breakfast. For a while, you focus on that, and that alone. Don't touch lunch or dinner. Just focus on breakfast.

At first, you might only succeed at eating the kind of breakfast that you want 2 out of 7 days. That's OK. Just try to beat that next week. **Practice involves a gradual build-up and gradual improvement. Not instant mastery.**

Once you find yourself eating the kind of breakfast that you want, 6-7 days per week, practice the next "skill." Maybe it's the skill of a better lunch. And use the same process for lunch as you did for breakfast.

What you'll find is that this process does take longer than crash dieting, but it's much more sustainable, and you feel much more successful doing it.

This is the process that I use with my clients when I'm doing nutritional counselling with them. There are a couple of additional resources that I share on habit change in the resource website associated with this book www.Mastering-Menopause.com.

Chapter 6

Exercise for Menopause

You might be in one of a few different categories:

- You've been a regular exerciser for years or decades, and when menopause hit, despite your exercise, you've noticed some changes in your body that you don't like.
- You've been exercising on and off, but now that your body is experiencing some changes that you don't like, you want to be more consistent with it.
- You've never exercised before, but you know that for your long-term health (and maybe vanity reasons), you should.
- You're not really a "gym person" but know that exercise is good for you. You just don't know what to do or how to do it.

Regardless of which category you're in, I have something for you in this chapter. We're going to cover:

- Whether postmenopausal women should exercise differently than premenopausal women.
- How exercise affects the hormone levels of postmenopausal women.
- Strength training exercise prescription.
- Cardio exercise prescription.

So without further ado, let's jump in.

How Exercise is Different Between Premenopausal and Postmenopausal Women

You know your body is different before and after menopause, but how different? There are 2 major differences that we'll cover at the end of this section, but there are also **a lot of similarities**.

Let's look at the similarities first.

In one study[11], researchers recruited one group of women between ages 20-30, and another group between ages 64-78. Both groups did the same exercise program (only leg extensions and leg curls) for 10 weeks.

The young women's muscle mass increased by 13%. In the older women, their muscle mass increased by 12%. A **negligible difference**.

In another study[2], women were divided into 3 different age groups:

- Under 45 years old
- 45-60
- Over 60

All 3 groups did the same strength training program. At the end of the 24-week study here were the results:

Age Group	Muscle Size	Muscle Strength
Under 45	Increased by 3.3%	Increased by 26%
45-60	Increased by 4.9%	Increased by 20%
Over 60	Increased by 4.1%	Increased by 26%

One meta-analysis[88] wanted to look at the extent to which lean body mass (that's not just muscle. Lean body mass is everything that's not fat, like bone, blood, skin, water, etc.) can increase in postmenopausal women over a 12-week period.

In this meta-analysis, women were doing predominantly full body workouts, for 3 sets of 8 reps, twice a week.

Over this duration, their **lean mass increased by 4.8%.** If that doesn't seem impressive to you, let's put that into perspective. As an example, if you're a 150-pound woman, with 33% body fat, it means you have 100 pounds of lean mass. Imagine **gaining 4.8 pounds of lean mass**. Not bad.

To put it into another perspective, **how much muscle mass do women lose after menopause**? One study[76] found that it's approximately 0.6% per year. **A gain of 4.8% in lean mass is almost like turning back the clock 8 years** (I say "almost" because again, muscle mass is only one component of lean mass. There are others. But presumably, if the 4.8% lean mass was gained because of strength training, it's largely – but not entirely – due to muscle gains).

This is from a research perspective. In research, the scientists must isolate variables. They have their participants just strength train without dietary changes.

In my experience with clients, we can get even greater improvements in lean mass by:

- Strength training 3-4 days per week, instead of the 2 in this meta-analysis[88].
- Optimizing the protein intake to the levels that I recommend in chapter 3.
- Doing it longer than 12 weeks. Studies are often limited by how much funding they have. If there's only enough funding for 12 weeks, then that's that.

In one study[15], researchers wanted to learn **by how much can muscle strength (not muscle mass) increase in postmenopausal women**. So they recruited women with an average age of 69 and had them do strength training for 12 weeks. The control group did nothing. After that period, **muscle strength improved by 28-115%** (depending on the muscle group), and there was a **20.1% increase in the size of a specific type of muscle fibres, called "fast-twitch muscle fibres."** There wasn't an increase in the size of slow-twitch muscle fibres (crash course: fast twitch muscle fibres have lots of speed/power, and very little endurance. Slow twitch muscle fibres are the opposite – lots of endurance, not much speed/power). There was (obviously) no increase in the muscle size of the control group.

Does that mean that people can maintain their strength into old age? Not really. You don't see 80-year-olds in the Olympics. But the relative degree of improvement appears to be similar between different ages. The absolute degree of improvement is different.

What do I mean by that? Let's say that we're comparing a 30-year-old woman to a 60-year-old woman. The 30-year-old can lift 100 pounds. The 60-year-old can lift 80 pounds. Both women increase their strength by 20%. That means that the 30-year-old increased her strength by 20 pounds. The 60-year-old increased her strength by 16 pounds. The relative improvement in strength is the same. The absolute is different.

Regardless, the fact that **improvement can be made so quickly at any age** should be very encouraging.

So as far as strength training is concerned, there are more similarities than differences. But as far as cardio is concerned, there is one key difference between premenopausal and postmenopausal women: **high intensity exercise is far superior to low intensity exercise for improving cardiovascular fitness**. While low intensity exercise is effective in premenopausal women, the **improvements in cardiovascular endurance in postmenopausal women from low and moderate-intensity exercise are minimal**.

Before going farther, since we'll be talking about cardio intensity a lot, let's give a few definitions:

- High intensity cardio: over 85% of the maximal heart rate (HRmax).
- Moderate intensity cardio: 60-85% of the HRmax.
- Low intensity cardio: under 60% HRmax.

    We'll talk about how to calculate your HRmax later in this chapter.

In one study[52], 16 premenopausal and 19 postmenopausal women were recruited. For 6 months, they did the exact same exercise program. They started at a frequency of 3 days per week, a duration of 20 minutes, and an intensity of 50% of their HRmax. Over a period of 4 weeks, the duration was increased to 40 minutes, and the intensity increased to 65%. The frequency stayed the same. Once participants reached 40 minutes and 65% intensity, they followed the same program for 5 more months.

After a total of 6 months, **the premenopausal women had an improvement of 13.3% in their endurance. The postmenopausal women had approximately a 1-2% improvement**. What a shame. You spend 6 months exercising, and almost nothing happens. You burned a few calories, but it didn't result in any improvements in your fitness.

Increase in endurance of premenopausal and postmenopausal women after 6 months of training

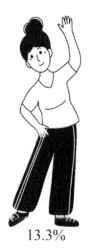 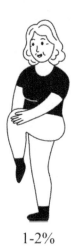

13.3%   1-2%

A meta-analysis[51] had slightly more encouraging results, but still not great – only a 5-8% improvement in aerobic capacity from cardio. However, in this meta-analysis, they analyzed all studies – low intensity, moderate, and high intensity. If you parse out the data and look at only the low and moderate intensity studies, you see the same conclusion: **minimal improvements in aerobic endurance**.

A couple of other ways of measuring cardiovascular fitness are the **resting heart rate** (RHR) and the **heart rate during exercise**.

In another study[22], that's exactly what was studied. It had a great design. The participants, who had an average age of 55 were randomly divided into 2 groups: low intensity and high intensity. Both groups exercised 3 times per week, for 50 minutes.

After this 10-week period, both groups completely stopped exercising for another 10 weeks, so that they'd lose all their progress on purpose. Then came a third 10-week period, where the groups switched – the group that was doing low intensity before was now doing high intensity, and vice versa.

What they found was that **both groups lowered their RHR by 5 beats per minute** (BPM). But there was a **clear superiority for the high intensity group in the exercise heart rate**. When both groups were tested at the same power output on the bike (they were pedalling at 120 Watts), the exercising heart rate of the low intensity group dropped by only 3 beats per minute (again, just about 2.6%). The exercising heart rate of the high intensity group dropped by 8.6 beats per minute (6.4%).

Reduction in Submaximal Heart Rate

High intensity group Low intensity group

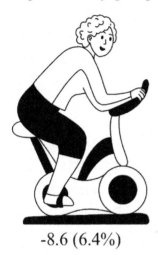 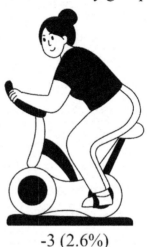

-8.6 (6.4%)   -3 (2.6%)

How this applies to real life: If you get winded climbing up the stairs, and you do low or moderate intensity cardio, you'll get winded going up the stairs just as much as if you weren't doing any cardio (a 2.6% drop in your exercise heart rate is barely noticeable). But if you do high intensity cardio, you'll actually feel that it's slightly easier going up the stairs.

Another study[61] backs up the case for high intensity cardio in postmenopausal women. In this study, the researchers recruited 40 premenopausal women (average age of 49), and 39 postmenopausal women (average age of 53). For 3 months, both groups followed the same exercise program – high intensity spinning classes, 3 times per week, for 1 hour.

At the end, the **premenopausal group improved their aerobic capacity by 8.8%. The postmenopausal group improved their aerobic capacity by 9.4%**.

A third study[60] compared high intensity exercise to no exercise. For 12 weeks, the exercise group did high intensity cardio 3 times per week, for 1 hour. At the end, the exercise group improved by 16%. The group that didn't exercise declined by 2%.

Basically, the research is fairly conclusive on this: **high intensity cardio is needed in order to improve cardiovascular endurance in postmenopausal women**. What's considered high intensity? In general, it's **over 85%** of your HRmax. How do you calculate your maximal heart rate? While there are lots of formulas out there, the most widely used formula is 220 minus your age.

So if hypothetically speaking, you're 60 years old, your maximal heart rate would be 160 beats per minute. You want to exercise at a minimum of 85% of 160, or 136 beats per minute. This will vary person-to-person, but this is a good starting point.

That's one major difference between premenopausal and postmenopausal women – **higher intensity cardio is necessary**. The other major difference, as discussed in chapter 2 is a **greater reliance on exercise for weight control after menopause**.

If you'll remember, **the main reason for weight gain after menopause is not a slowdown of the metabolism**. If that ever happens, it's only very minor, according to a very large study[70] Research[71] shows that **the primary reason for weight gain during and after menopause is a reduction in involuntary activity** (like fidgeting).

If involuntary activity drops, we have to compensate for that with voluntary activity - exercise. It's a cliché by now that when it comes to weight loss, it's 80% diet and 20% exercise. Not the case for postmenopausal women. The exercise portion plays a much greater role in weight control for postmenopausal women. One study[54] of 34,079 women showed that **the women who gained the least weight after menopause are those that exercised the most**... as if we needed a study to tell us that.

When it comes to exercise post-menopause, **frequency trumps everything**. Whether it's formal exercise, where you're sweating it out in the gym and going to fitness classes, or just movement that isn't purposeful exercise (like walking, skiing, a game of tennis, etc.), it's better to be active 4-7 days a week.

How Exercise Affects the Hormone Levels of Postmenopausal Women

One of the biggest reasons for changes in health risks after menopause is the general drops in hormone levels. Can you change your hormone levels (and therefore, presumably risk of chronic conditions) with exercise? You can!

In one study[65] of 182 postmenopausal women, they were divided into 2 groups. One group exercised for a year, and the other group didn't. At the end of 1 year, here were the changes in their hormone levels:

Group	Estradiol	Estrone	Testosterone
Didn't exercise	Decreased by 24.4%	Decreased by 13.9%	Decreased by ~10%
Exercised, lost <2% body fat	Decreased by 24.4%	Decreased by 13.9%	Decreased by ~10%
Exercised, lost >2% body fat	Decreased by 11.7%	Decreased by 23.7%	Decreased by ~10%

Here are the Cliff's notes:

- Estradiol was higher in the group that exercised and lost more than 2% body fat.
- Estrone was higher in the groups that didn't exercise and those that exercised but lost less than 2% body fat.
- No matter whether the women exercised or not, **all the hormones decreased regardless**. Exercise only affected the extent of the decrease, but not whether or not hormone levels decreased.

In another study[62] of 12 months, 173 overweight/obese sedentary women, between ages 50 and 75 were divided into 2 groups:

- Exercise: 45+ minutes of moderate-intensity cardio (60-75% of the maximal heart rate), 5 days a week.
- Control: no exercise.

Both groups were asked to maintain their usual diets.

Here were the results after a year:

Exercise/Control	Body Fat Status	Hormone	Change
Exercise	Gained	Estrone	Increased 5.8%
Control	Gained	Estrone	Increased 4.5%
Exercise	Unchanged	Estrone	Increased 14.4%
Control	Unchanged	Estrone	Increased 5.7%
Exercise	Lost 0.5-2%	Estrone	Decreased 1.6%
Control	Lost 0.5-2%	Estrone	Increased 3.8%
Exercise	Lost more than 2%	Estrone	Decreased 11.9%
Control	Lost more than 2%	Estrone	Decreased 3.6%
Exercise	Gained	Free Estradiol	Increased 5.7%

Control	Gained	Free Estradiol	Decreased 5.7%
Exercise	Unchanged	Free Estradiol	Increased 9.1%
Control	Unchanged	Free Estradiol	Decreased 2.1%
Exercise	Lost 0.5-2%	Free Estradiol	Decreased 9.8%
Control	Lost 0.5-2%	Free Estradiol	Increased 2.3%
Exercise	Lost more than 2%	Free Estradiol	Decreased 16.7%
Control	Lost more than 2%	Free Estradiol	Increased 2.2%

To summarize, there's plenty of research on how exercise affects hormone levels in postmenopausal women. Unfortunately, researchers, being geeks who like to look inside test tubes, never wonder to whom the specimen in the test tube belongs. So they measure hormone levels, but never extend it to ask the participants how it affected their symptoms.

We can only theorize how changing hormone levels affect menopausal symptoms, but without questionnaires, we simply don't know. Unfortunately at the present time, there's almost no research on how exercise affects menopausal symptoms.

Fortunately, there's plenty of research on how exercise affects disease risk in postmenopausal women. The short answer: depending on the type of exercise, it reduces the risk of a lot of conditions. The long answer – I elaborate on it in 3 books that I've published on the topic:

- *Osteoporosis Reversal Secrets*
- *High Blood Pressure Reversal Secrets*
- *Type 2 Diabetes Reversal Secrets*

The first chapter of each of these books has been made available to you at www.Mastering-Menopause.com.

Shortly after this book that you're reading right now, I'll also be publishing a book on osteoarthritis, so if you want to relieve joint pain from wear-and-tear, perhaps it's already out at the time you're reading this.

Strength Training Exercise Prescription

Now you know the ins and outs of how exercise is different before menopause vs. after, as well as how exercise affects the levels of different hormones. But how should you exercise? What should you do, on a practical level?

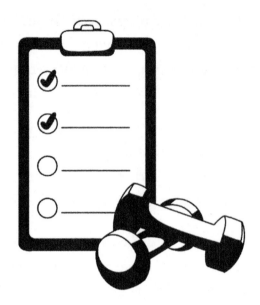

While exercise program design is a complex subject, and there are several variables that enter the equation. In this section, I'll give you some general principles, based on 3 common goals. As for specific exercises, we'll cover that in the following section.

Goal: Fat Loss

The purpose of strength training for someone looking to lose body fat is not gaining muscle. The purpose is **preserving muscle**. When you're losing body fat, some muscle loss can happen. The amount of muscle lost can be substantial if you're not strength training, and you're on a low-protein diet. But this can be dramatically minimized if you're strength training, and you're on a normal-protein diet (not even a high-protein diet).

"But I want to gain muscle and lose fat", I can hear you thinking. Unfortunately **you can't do both at the same time**. Why not? Because to lose fat, you need to eat fewer calories than it takes to maintain your weight. If you want to gain muscle, you need to eat more calories than it takes to maintain your weight. Since you can't have more and less at the same time, **you have to prioritize**. Which one do you want first? Once you've accomplished that one, you switch to the other one.

If you're wondering "which one *should* I do first"? My general rule is **if a woman has over about 30% body fat, I recommend fat loss first**, muscle gain second. **If a woman is under 22% body fat, I recommend muscle gain first**, and fat loss second. If a woman is between 22% and 30%, her choice.

Now, when it comes to a strength training prescription, we want to know 5 different elements:

1. **Frequency**: how many days per week.
2. **Intensity**: how hard.
3. **Volume**: how many sets and reps.
4. **Full body workouts or body part splits** (where you do different body parts on different days).
5. **Straight sets, circuit sets, or supersets** (straight sets are where you do an exercise, rest, and repeat the same exercise again. Circuit sets are when you complete 1 set of each of the exercises, before repeating all the exercises for a 2nd set. Supersets are where you pair up 2 different exercises. You perform 1 set of the first exercise, and 1 set of the 2nd exercise. Then rest. That's one superset. You perform the prescribed number of sets before moving on to the next group of 2 exercises).

So here's your strength training prescription for fat loss:

105

- **Frequency**: 2-3 days per week.
- **Intensity**: use a weight that gets you close to muscular failure (the point at which you can't do any more repetitions).
- **Volume**: 2-3 sets of 15-20 repetitions.
- **Full body workouts** (the actual exercises are coming up).
- **Circuit sets or supersets**.

Goal: Strength Without Muscle Mass

If you want to gain strength without gaining muscle mass, here's your exercise prescription:

- **Frequency**: 2-4 days per week.
- **Intensity**: use a weight that keeps you 3-4 repetitions from muscular failure.
- **Volume**: 3-5 sets of 3-5 repetitions.
- **Full body workouts** (the actual exercises are coming up).
- **Circuit sets, supersets or straight sets**. They all work for this purpose.

Goal: Muscle Mass and Strength

If you don't mind gaining a few pounds of muscle, here's your exercise prescription:

- **Frequency**: 2-4 days per week.
- **Intensity**: use a weight that keeps you 0-2 repetitions from muscular failure.

- **Number of sets per muscle, per week**: 8-10. So if you're strength training twice per week, you'd be doing 4-5 sets per muscle per workout. If you're strength training three times per week, you'd be doing about 3 sets per muscle, per workout. If you're strength training four times per week, you'd be doing 2-3 sets per muscle, per workout.
- **Number of repetitions**: anywhere from 5-20. As long as you're **coming very close to muscular failure**.
- **Full body workouts** (the actual exercises are coming up).
- **Circuit sets, supersets or straight sets**. They all work for this purpose, but straight sets will take a lot more time.

Gym Exercises

You now know the exercise prescriptions for different goals. But which exercises do you do? That's what we'll cover in this section.

The reason that I left this section for the end is because there are no "fat loss exercises" and a different set of exercises for muscle gain, and another different set of exercises for diabetes, or high blood pressure, etc. The exercise may be the same. What changes is the weight, the sets, repetitions, and frequency. For instance, squats done for 3 sets of 15-20 reps might be a fat loss exercise. But squats done for 5 sets of 3-5 reps might be a strength exercise. The exercise is the same – but the sets, reps and weight are different.

Here are some of my favourite exercises to use if you have access to a gym:

- One-legged deadlifts
- Lat pulldowns

- Barbell overhead press
- Squats
- Seated rows
- Incline pushups
- Calf raises.

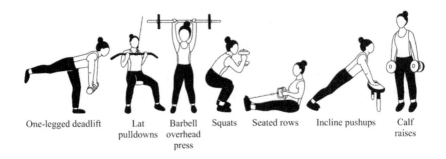

One-legged deadlift | Lat pulldowns | Barbell overhead press | Squats | Seated rows | Incline pushups | Calf raises

Simply pick which of the above goals you're interested in, and plug the exercises into the right frequency, intensity, volume and format (circuits, supersets or straight sets).

If you want to see videos of these exercises, they're available for you at www.Mastering-Menopause.com.

Home Exercises

If you don't have access to a gym or you're not a "gym person", here are some home exercises. The only assumption I'm making is that at home, **you have dumbbells and resistance bands**. In my experience, most women have very light dumbbells at home, like 15 pounds and less. Most women seriously underestimate their strength (even sedentary postmenopausal women). Initially, I recommend **getting dumbbells up to 50 pounds**. If you think you can't do that yet, it's because you're likely thinking of biceps curls.

The biceps are a lot weaker than the quads (front of the thighs) or glutes (buttocks). **Your biceps might not be able to handle a heavy weight, but your legs and butt probably can**. So don't be shy about getting those 50-pound dumbbells.

Anyways, with that out of the way, here are your at-home exercises using just dumbbells and resistance bands:

- One-legged deadlifts
- Banded lat pulldowns
- Dumbbell overhead press
- Squats
- Banded seated rows
- Incline pushups
- Calf raises.

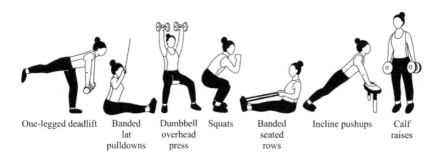

One-legged deadlift · Banded lat pulldowns · Dumbbell overhead press · Squats · Banded seated rows · Incline pushups · Calf raises

Yes, there's a lot of overlap between the gym exercises and the at-home exercises. That's because I want you to be able to **do the exercises anywhere**. I don't want to give you exercises with highly specialized equipment that only one gym has, but no others.

Again, if you want to see videos of these exercises, they're available to you at www.Mastering-Menopause.com.

Cardio Exercise Prescription

Before we jump into the really important part, let's answer the question of "**Which machine should I do**"? Because that part is actually not all that important. The machine itself doesn't matter. Whether you use a treadmill (or run outdoors), an elliptical, a bike, swimming, rowing, etc. doesn't matter. **What really matters is the variables we're about to discuss** (frequency, intensity, number of intervals, etc.).

So either pick your favourite cardio exercise and stick with it, or if you like/hate everything equally, alternate machines. There are a few different ways of alternating:

- **By day**: one day you do one machine, the next day, you do a different machine.
- **By duration**: one 10-minute segment you do one machine, the next 10-minute segment you do a different machine.
- **By week or month**.

With that out of the way, let's talk about what really matters. Just as there are parameters to strength training (frequency, intensity, volume, etc.), there are also parameters to cardio. They are:

- **Frequency**: how many days per week.
- **Intensity**: this is based on your pulse. How close are you working to your maximal heart rate.
- **Number of intervals**.
- **Interval duration**: if you're doing interval training (where you're going hard for a period of time, followed by easy for another period of time), this is the duration of the "hard" part of the interval.

- **Workout duration**: more relevant to steady cardio, as opposed to interval training.

You'll see lots of books with duration recommendations based on time. Here's the thing: **time is arbitrary. It's how your body responds to time that really matters.** For example, one woman might do a 1-minute interval at 6 miles per hour, and at the end of 1 minute, she has a pulse of 150 beats per minute. Another woman, of the same age and weight might do the exact same interval but have a pulse of only 135 beats per minute. Did that workout affect both women the same way? No.

Likewise, the first time you did a 1-minute interval, at a speed of 6 miles per hour (for instance), you might have had a pulse of 150 beats per minute. After a few weeks, you did the same workout, but now have a pulse of 142 beats per minute. The absolute intensity (speed, interval duration, etc.) might be the same. But the relative intensity (how your body handled it) is different.

Furthermore, there are **day-to-day variations in the way you feel and perform**. Some days, your pulse recovers in 90 seconds, and other days, your pulse recovers in 75 seconds.

There are even **interval-to-interval variations in your pulse**. When you're fresh, you recover faster. Towards the end of your workout, you recover slower. So if you were to give recommendations based on an arbitrary recovery time in between intervals, the early intervals are easy, and the later intervals are very difficult.

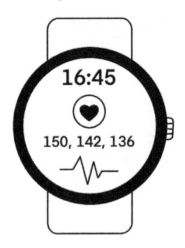

Hence the need to give recommendations based on pulse, as opposed to time. With pulse, you'll adjust the difficulty to meet the required pulse. **Pulse-based recommendations solve many of the problems with time-based recommendations**.

So here is a sample, 3-day-per-week cardio workout:

Day 1

- **Interval duration**: 60 seconds
- **Intensity**: 85-90% of your HRmax
- **Number of intervals**: 4-12
- **When to start the next interval**: when your pulse comes down to 65% of your HRmax

The goal is to **reach the required pulse as early in the interval as possible**. If you need to adjust the speed/resistance throughout the interval, that's OK.

Day 2

- **Interval duration:** 30 seconds
- **Intensity:** 85-90% of your HRmax
- **Number of intervals:** 6-18
- **When to start the next interval:** when your pulse comes down to 65% of your HRmax

Day 3

- **Interval duration:** 15 seconds
- **Intensity:** 90-95% of your top speed
- **Number of intervals:** 8-30
- **When to start the next interval:** when your pulse comes down to 65% of your HRmax

With 15-second intervals, you can't give interval intensity recommendations based on pulse, because the elevation in pulse is a bit delayed. Throughout all 15 seconds, the pulse will be climbing. The pulse will actually peak 10-15 seconds **after** you finish the interval.

One note I should make on measuring your pulse – remember how in chapter 3 (nutrition), we talked about the atrocious accuracy of nutrition tracking apps? Unfortunately the same thing applies to most heart rate monitors on the market. If a heart rate monitor does not have a chest strap, it's not accurate. They're all bad – Fitbits, Apple watches, Whoop straps, Oura rings, etc. **Those that have a chest strap are indeed accurate**. Or, you can always go "old school", and measure your pulse at your wrist, or at your throat (carotid), and that has great accuracy.

Earlier, I mentioned all the advantages of using heart rate to guide your cardio workouts, but there is one big downside: complexity. If you're not used to this method, it seems complex. I get it. When you read it, it's complex, but try it over a period of 3-5 workouts, and once it's applied in your workouts, you'll start to understand it much better than just reading it.

Chapter 7

Perimenopausal Aches and Pains

Several of my clients have reported that in their younger years, they were very active and athletic, but now, in their 40s, 50s and 60s, even a reduced level of activity/exercise causes:

- Fatigue that takes longer to recover from.
- Minor injuries here and there – tendonitis, and others.
- Exaggerated **soreness** – disproportionate to the intensity of the workout.

What's going on? That's what we'll cover in this chapter.

How Do Estrogen Levels Impact Injury Risk in Women?

In one study[17], researchers removed the ovaries from rats (thereby really diminishing their estrogen levels), and assessed their recovery from a rat's everyday life, along with injury risk.

What they found was:

- 14 days after ovary removal, the rats had a **slower recovery**.
- During days 7-14, the number of **injured fibres increased**.
- After 14 days, the rats were given estrogen, to bring their levels back to what they were before the removal of their ovaries, and the **damaged fibres healed**.

So why does estrogen reduce the risk of injuries? There are a few theories:

1. Estrogen impacts muscle size and strength. Less estrogen, less muscle. If there's less muscle, **the stress from exercise that used to go into muscles now goes into tendons and ligaments**.

2. Estrogen stabilizes what's called the "extracellular matrix" (or ECM). What is the ECM? It's a group of "support structures" that help stabilize cells. What are those structures? Things like collagen, different minerals, and others. Different structures (bones, muscles, etc.) have different compositions of the ECM. **Less estrogen means less "supporting structures" for muscles, tendons and ligaments**.

3. Estrogen can act as an antioxidant, and decrease the damage that muscles, tendons and ligaments sustain.

To test these theories, in one study[39], researchers gave postmenopausal women enough estrogen to bring them up to premenopausal levels. What they found was that:

- Collagen synthesis improved by 47%.
- Grip strength improved.
- Muscle mass increased a bit.

The effects on grip and muscle mass were fairly minor, but **the effects on collagen synthesis in the tendons was quit**

significant. The researchers pointed out that muscle mass and strength improve a lot more with strength training than with estrogen replacement therapy.

Obviously, this is not a book about hormone replacement therapy (HRT), as I'm not qualified to advise on that, but in the previous chapter, you learned how exercise affects hormone levels. In the next chapter, you'll also learn which supplements may help increase estrogen.

How do Progesterone Levels Impact Injury Risk in Women?

In the perimenopausal period, it's not just estrogen that declines, but other hormones as well. Namely, progesterone, testosterone and, in some women, thyroid too.

So how does progesterone impact injury risk in women? While progesterone alone is not studied nearly as extensively as estrogen, one study[57] found that **progesterone really doesn't have much of an impact on injury risk in postmenopausal women**.

What did the researchers do in that one?

They divided the participants into 5 groups: 1 placebo group, 2 groups who received only estrogen (no progesterone), at 2 different doses, and 2 more groups who received both estrogen and progesterone (same progesterone dose, but different estrogen doses).

What they found, which is consistent with previous studies, is that increasing estrogen after menopause does decrease injury risk.

But when estrogen was raised, and progesterone was raised as well, there was no additional decrease in injury risk.

So in a nutshell: **progesterone doesn't appear to have much of an impact on injury risk in the postmenopausal years**. Not to say it's not important. It is. But just looking at it through the lens of its impact on tendons and ligaments, it doesn't have much of an impact. It may impact other health parameters, like your heart, brain, skin, etc., but since this chapter is about injury risk, we're really looking at muscles, tendons, and ligaments.

How Do Testosterone Levels Impact Injury Risk in Women?

Similar to progesterone, testosterone is not studied very well in postmenopausal women (at least when it comes to injury risk). However, there are a couple of studies to go by, though the ultimate conclusion (as you see so often in research) is we don't have the full picture, so more research is necessary.

With that disclaimer out of the way, let's examine what the research has to say.

It's been well-established[38] that **testosterone affects women's muscle mass**. We also know[24] that it also **affects women's bone density**. But how does testosterone affect women's tendons and ligaments? That's not as clear.

One study[38] did show that women's tendons have receptors for testosterone. What that means is that testosterone affects women's tendons. It's theorized that it **improves tendon stiffness**. Tendon stiffness is a good thing. A stiff tendon is a more injury-resistant tendon.

So we know that testosterone affects women's tendons. What about their ligaments (side note: most people don't know the difference between tendons and ligaments. So I'll give you a quick lesson right now. Tendons connect muscle to bone. Ligaments connect bone to bone. You're welcome.). One study[87] found that **women with lower testosterone levels are more prone to ACL tears** (that's one of the ligaments inside your knee). Another study[59] found **lower ACL stiffness in women with lower testosterone**. Lower ACL stiffness typically means a higher rate of ACL tears.

As we know from the previous chapter, exercise doesn't impact testosterone levels in postmenopausal women. So whether you should be increasing your testosterone levels or not should be a conversation between you and your doctor or endocrinologist.

What Can You Do?

So we know that some hormones have a definite impact on injury and recovery in perimenopausal and postmenopausal women. Other hormones have no impact, and some hormones, we just don't know.

But what are non-hormonal ways to decrease the risk of injury?

The non-hormonal factors are **protein, sleep, and collagen supplementation**. In chapter 3, we discussed protein – simply follow the protein recommendations from that chapter. Sleep, we'll discuss in chapter 9.

Non-hormonal ways to decrease the risk of injury

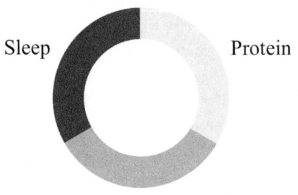

Sleep   Protein

Collagen supplementation

As for collagen supplementation, the research is very limited in postmenopausal women, so right now, we have to rely on research from other populations (like men and premenopausal women). In one study[46], men were divided into 2 groups:

- Collagen (5 grams/day of specific collagen peptides)
- Placebo

After 14 weeks, the **collagen group increased their muscle thickness by 7.3%.** The placebo group only increased it by 2.7%.

In another study[74], 20 people (a mix of men and women, with an average age of 44) were divided into 2 groups:

- Group 1: collagen first, for 3 months, and then placebo for 3 months.
- Group 2: placebo first, for 3 months, and then collagen for 3 months.

To be eligible to participate in the study, the people had to be runners who've had to stop running due to injuries.

In group 1, **60% of the runners were able to return to running in 3 months**. In group 2, only 30% of the runners were able to return to running in 3 months. After 6 months, 70% of the runners in group 1 were able to return to running, and 50% of the runners in group 2 were able to return to running.

So based on the current research, it appears that collagen is effective in preventing injuries, and speeding up recovery from them. But the devil is in the details. Both studies we looked at used **specific collagen peptides (SCPs), and a dose of 5 grams per day**. Lots of women take type 3 collagen for their hair, skin and nails. But tendons and ligaments are not made of type 3 collagen. So make sure you're taking the right type and dose of collagen for tendons and ligaments.

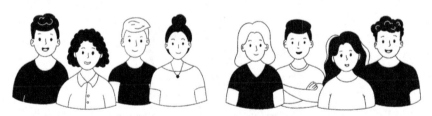

Group 1: collagen first for 3 months, then placebo for 3 months	Group 2: placebo first for 3 months, then collagen for 3 months
60% of the runners were able to return to running in 3 months	30% of the runners were able to return to running in 3 months
70% of the runners were able to return to running after 6 months	50% of the runners were able to return to running after 6 months

Chapter 8

Supplements for Menopause

Some people are taking boatloads of supplements, constantly looking for the magic pill. Others are completely skeptical of supplements, thinking they're just a hoax. The truth is somewhere in the middle. But make no mistake about it – **there are some very potent, proven supplements out there that can help you improve your menopause symptoms**. Likewise, there are also tons of supplements that are unproven, and by the end of this chapter, you'll know what works, what doesn't, and what we don't know.

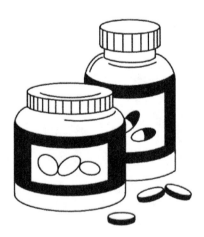

Here's what we'll cover in this chapter:

- Two myths about supplements.

- Three reasons why I REALLY like supplements.

- How to find the right dose.

- 4 effective supplements to improve menopausal symptoms.

- 2 ineffective supplements for improving menopausal symptoms – even though they're often included in menopause formulas.

- 7 unproven supplements.

- How to combine supplements.

- Why ineffective and unproven ingredients are often added to supplements.

But before we get to it, I have to make the obligatory disclaimer: I don't know you. I don't know your health status, what other supplements and medications you are taking, and other pertinent factors. So before you start taking any of the supplements in this chapter, **speak to a pharmacist first**. A lot of people make the mistake of thinking "supplements are natural; therefore they can't do any harm." And boy, are they wrong. Mixing some supplements with some medications can have negative effects in some people.

So again, speak to a pharmacist before you start taking any of these supplements.

With that disclaimer out of the way, let's get to it!

Supplement Myths

Myth #1: Supplements Don't Work

For someone to believe this one, they'd really have to completely ignore the mountains of research done over the decades that supplements do work. That's not to say that every single supplement on the market works. And that's not to say that every supplement works for 100% of people. But to make a blanket statement that there isn't a single supplement out there that works is just plain false.

Then there's the cousin – "**it's just a placebo effect**." First of all, no it's not. In double-blind, placebo-controlled studies, the term "placebo-controlled" means that one group of participants in the study are getting a placebo, and the other is getting the real supplement, and consistently, **the right supplement outperforms the placebo**. Therefore it can't be the placebo effect.

Second of all, even if it was a placebo effect, so what? The placebo effect is a real, measurable effect. If your menopause symptoms improved, whether due to something real, or something in your mind, who cares about the reason? You're forgetting the main point – **your symptoms improved**!

Myth #2: You Have to Make Dietary Changes First

False again. In most studies, researchers specifically tell participants not to make any dietary changes when they're taking supplements. Why? Because if you start taking a supplement, and you change your diet at the same time, you don't know if the effect was caused by the supplement, by the diet, or both.

And **even in the absence of any dietary changes, some supplements work**. Again, that's not to say that every supplement works (we'll cover what works and what doesn't later in this chapter), but those that do work do so in the absence of any dietary changes.

Three Reasons Why I Really Like Supplements

As you can tell, I'm a big fan of supplements. There are 3 reasons for this. In no particular order:

Reason #1: Effectiveness

As I mentioned in the previous section, the supplements that work do so in their own right, in the absence of any dietary changes. Would you get an additive effect if you combined them with changes in exercise and nutrition? Sure. But you still get anywhere from a moderate to a large effect on your symptoms without any other changes.

Reason #2: Compliance

If you've ever been on a diet before, you know that dietary changes are hard. If you've been eating a certain way for 40, 50, 60 years or more, it's very hard to change those long-standing habits.

But taking a pill, powder or liquid? That's easy! Most people have near-100% compliance with that. Whereas dietary changes (given that 80-95% of people who lose weight regain it), don't have anywhere near the same compliance level.

Reason #3: Speed of Effect

Some supplements work quickly (in a matter of days), and other supplements take 3 months of taking them regularly to have any effect. But even if a supplement takes 3 months to work, that's better than not working.

How to Find the Right Supplement Dose

With any supplement, you want to make sure you're taking a dose high enough that it's effective, but low enough that it doesn't cause any adverse effects.

There are a couple of factors that go into figuring out the optimal dose for you:

Factor #1: **your own bodyweight**. The more you weigh, the more of a dose you need.

Factor #2: your **personal reactivity** to it. Some people are highly responsive to supplements, and others aren't.

To figure out the right dose for you, here's a step-by-step process you should use:

Step 1: don't take any supplements for menopause just yet (if you're taking supplements for other reasons, keep taking them). Just take an inventory of your symptoms for 1 week. Either create your own or download the one I've provided for you at www.Mastering-Menopause.com. You're going to be using this baseline to see if the supplements you try are effective.

<u>Step 2</u>: **start at the dose that it says on the label** of whatever supplement you're taking. Stay at that dose for 2 weeks. Note if it had the desirable effect (did it improve your symptoms?).

<u>Step 3</u>: **raise the dose by the smallest possible increment** for another 2 weeks. Note if after an additional 2 weeks the effect increased, or stayed the same. If the effect stayed the same, go back to the dose used in step 1. If the effect increased, move on to step 5.

<u>Step 4</u>: keep repeating step 3 until either the effect has maxed out (no larger drops in symptoms despite larger doses), or you've reached the maximal safe dose.

<u>Step 5</u>: after about 1-2 months, try reducing the dose by the smallest possible increment. If the symptoms are unchanged after 2 weeks at the lower dose, reduce it again by the smallest possible increment. However, if the symptoms increased after you reduced the dose, raise it back up again.

Effective Supplements

Now, we get to the fun part: the supplements that work. The supplements listed here have been shown to work in multiple studies in humans. I emphasize "in humans" because a lot of supplements go to market prematurely. They're shown to work in either mice/rats, or petri dishes. But not people. Each supplement listed in this section has been shown to work in people, across more than 1 study.

<u>Black Cohosh (AKA Cimicifuga Racemosa AKA Actaea Racemosa)</u>

One meta-analysis[78] showed that **black cohosh reduced hot flashes by 31.5%** more than placebo. It also **reduced somatic symptoms (headaches, joint and muscle aches) by 41.8%** more than placebo. But it had no effect on anxiety or depression.

Another meta-analysis[13] concluded that "efficacy of iCR [black cohosh] was **comparable to low-dose transdermal estradiol or tibolone**. Yet, due to its better tolerability, iCR had a significantly better benefit–risk profile than tibolone."

One study[58] showed **no difference between low dose (39 mg) and high dose (127.3 mg) of black cohosh** in women beyond the early stages of menopause. But there was a difference for women in early menopause. They did better with the higher dose.

How it works: interestingly enough, it's not by raising estrogen levels. One study[75] found that it modulates neurotransmitter activity (brain chemicals, like serotonin, dopamine, GABA) in postmenopausal women. These neurotransmitters affect mood, temperature regulation and sleep.

Upper limit: while the dose at which toxicity symptoms are experienced is unknown, the highest dose given in research[58] is 127.3 mg.

Symptoms of toxicity (comparable to placebo, according to this study[13]):

- Nausea and vomiting
- Headache
- Hypotension
- Liver damage

Soy Isoflavones

- One meta-analysis[63] showed that soy isoflavones **reduced hot flash frequency by 20.6%, and severity by 26.2%** more than placebo.
- No effect on mood swings[83].
- Effects on fatigue: unknown.
- Vaginal dryness is reduced by 31%[68].

How it works: One systematic review[68] showed that it's **anti-inflammatory** (reduces TNF-alpha and IL-6. These are markers of inflammation). A second mechanism of action is that soy isoflavones behave both like weak estrogens, as well as antiestrogens (the estrogen story is actually very complex. There are different estrogen receptors in different tissues. Some estrogen receptors have a proliferative effect, and other estrogen receptors negate the proliferative effect. I told you it's complex. If you want to dive into this in more detail, just check out the research associated with this section).

Upper limit: unknown, but the typical dose used in research is 50-100 mg/day for 12 weeks, however that's a combination of both dietary soy isoflavones, as well as supplemental.

Symptoms of toxicity:

- Constipation
- Nausea
- Bloating
- Allergic reaction (rash, itching)

Sage Leaf (AKA salvia officinalis)

I was debating whether to put sage leaf in this section or in the section on unproven supplements. The reason for this debate is that there's very little research. There are only 2 studies that I'm aware of (in humans). But since it meets our criteria of having at least 1 study in humans, I decided to include it in this section.

One study[99] showed that sage leaf **decreases both the severity and frequency of hot flashes** (in that study, it was taken for 12 weeks). The group that received sage leaf **lowered their hot flash severity by 40%, and the frequency by 73%**. In comparison, the control group lowered the severity of their hot flashes by 12%, and the frequency by 9%.

Another study[94] showed a **31% difference in menopausal symptoms** between the group on sage leaf and the group on placebo, after 4 weeks. In this study, all menopausal symptoms were studied (somatic, urogenital, and psychological).

How it works: sage leaf controls neurotransmitters responsible for thermoregulation (acetylcholine and norepinephrine).

Upper limit: unknown, but research uses 100 mg, 3 times a day.

Symptoms of toxicity:

- Vomiting
- Tachycardia
- Salivation
- Vertigo

Red Clover

One systematic review[49] found that red clover extract **reduced the frequency by 1.73 hot flashes per day**.

Another systematic review[32] found that red clover **reduced the frequency of hot flashes by 5 per day**. The higher the number of hot flashes a woman had, the greater the reduction. But there's less of an effect on psychological, sexual, and sleeping symptoms of menopause.

How it Works: one mechanism of action is that it has estrogenic activity. Another mechanism is that it has anti-inflammatory and anti-oxidative effects (reference[35]).

Upper limit: unknown, but the dose used in research is typically 40-80 mg/day.

Symptoms of toxicity:

- Bloating
- Diarrhea

Ineffective Supplements

Now you are aware of all the supplements that are proven to improve menopausal symptoms (at the time of this writing). There are also lots of supplements said to improve menopausal symptoms, but either largely don't do so or don't do so at all. That doesn't mean they have no benefit for other reasons, but as far as menopausal symptoms are concerned, they are proven ineffective (although that doesn't stop a lot of supplement manufacturers from putting them into menopause formulas, and claiming they work, despite evidence to the contrary).

Dong Quay (AKA Angelica Sinensis)

Dong quay is a darling in the menopause supplement world, but for no good reason. In one study[43], 71 postmenopausal women received either placebo or dong quay for 24 weeks. Those who got dong quay got a dose of 0.5 mg/kg. It wasn't effective in relieving menopausal symptoms.

In another study[25], women who took 5g/day of dong quay for 24 weeks showed no changes in menopausal symptoms.

Chaste Tree Berry (AKA Vitex)

This is another darling of the menopause supplement world that is unjustified. One systematic review[53] found that it wasn't effective in relieving menopausal symptoms, at various different doses.

If you're wondering "Why are ineffective ingredients added to menopause supplements, with the claim that they relieve symptoms?", we'll address that later in this chapter. Stay tuned.

Unproven Supplements

Very often, people confuse "unproven" with "ineffective." But they're not the same. Ineffective means "it doesn't work." But **"unproven" means "we don't know if it works."** Either studies haven't been done, or the studies had methodological flaws that make conclusions about effectiveness very difficult.

Fortunately, you don't care about averages – you care about you. You can do your own "study" on yourself. My first instinct with clients is to recommend what's proven and has a high degree of efficacy. But if you want to try the unproven supplements, go for it (after a conversation with a pharmacist, of course). You will learn about how these supplements affect your body, in less time than it takes to conduct a study.

Gamma Oryzanol

One study[30] showed relief from anxiety, irritability, depression and insomnia. Unfortunately that study didn't include any information on the dose used, or by how much the symptoms were reduced.

Other than that, there's no research that I'm aware of on dosages, toxicity, or safety.

How it might work:

- Releases neurotransmitters that help with stress management.
- Has anti-inflammatory and anti-oxidative effects, which may help with the physical complaints of menopause.

Upper limit: unknown

Side effects:

- Dry mouth

- Sleepiness
- Hot flashes
- Irritability
- Light-headedness

Hesperidin

Hesperidin has no available research on it whatsoever for the purpose of menopausal symptom relief. There is some minor research on hesperidin for other conditions (like diabetes, high cholesterol, cancer, etc.), but even in those conditions, the research is really light.

For menopause, there's no information on dosage, toxicity, side effects, mechanisms or anything else.

Inositol

Inositol is another supplement with no research on how it affects menopausal symptoms. There's just a single study[34] on how it affects metabolic syndrome in menopausal and postmenopausal women but it was combined with diet. The group receiving diet + inositol had great improvements in metabolic syndrome (17% drop in fasting blood glucose, 69% drop in fasting insulin, 20% drop in total cholesterol, 25% increase in HDL, 21% drop in triglycerides). The group doing the diet + placebo had smaller improvements in metabolic syndrome (4% drop in fasting blood glucose, 14% drop in fasting insulin, 7% drop in total cholesterol, 1% rise in HDL, 3% drop in triglycerides).

So we know that for metabolic syndrome in menopausal and postmenopausal women it's pretty good. But as for its effect specifically on menopausal symptoms, we don't know. Outside of that application, inositol is actually my most frequently recommended supplement for PCOS (polycystic ovarian syndrome).

Upper limit: 12 grams/day

Side effects:

- Nausea
- Stomach pain
- Fatigue
- Headache
- Dizziness

Multivitamins

I frequently recommend multivitamins in situations where either food intake is low (like someone purposely cutting tons of calories temporarily), or absorption is bad (in conditions like Inflammatory Bowel Disease, Crohn's, colitis, etc.).

However, as far as menopausal symptoms are concerned, there's **no research about how multivitamins affect them**.

Also, unlike the other ingredients in this section, multivitamins are not one standard thing. Different multis vary widely in their composition. Because of that, no recommendations for dosages, or side effects can be given.

Fish Oil

I frequently recommend fish oil for lowering high blood pressure, improving depression, decreasing the pain of osteoarthritis, and other health goals/conditions. However, the relief of menopausal symptoms is not one of those health goals/conditions.

Currently, there is **no research on how fish oil affects menopausal symptoms**.

Upper limit: unknown.

Symptoms of toxicity:

- Oil leakage out of anus
- Bleeding
- Diarrhea
- Insomnia
- Indigestion
- Vomiting

Hop Extract

We know from the nutrition chapter that beer is great for reducing menopausal symptoms. So it stands to reason that hop extract (the part of the beer thought to be helpful for symptoms) would also be helpful for menopause.

Unfortunately, there's just a single study exploring that. And our criteria for including something in either the effective or ineffective section is that there's more than one study. In this case, there isn't. And the one study[42] that does exist found that both the placebo group and the hop extract group lowered their symptoms by almost the same degree.

How it might work: it's estrogenic.

Upper limit: 300 mg/day

Toxicity symptoms:

- Sleepiness
- Slow breathing

Evening Primrose Oil (AKA Oenothera Biennis)

The evidence on EPO (that's evening primrose oil for our purposes, not erythropoietin) is very mixed. One meta-analysis[18] found no difference between EPO and placebo when it comes to vasomotor symptoms (hot flashes, night sweats, etc.).

But one study[79] did find an **improvement in psychological symptoms**. In this study, 100 menopausal women were given either EPO (1 g/day) or placebo for 4 weeks. At the end of the study, the group that received EPO had a **73% reduction in psychological symptoms**. The placebo group had no change. Seems promising, but it is just one study. No other studies have replicated these results.

How it might work: EPO is rich in gamma linoleic acid, which is a type of an unsaturated fat. Depression is associated with having a low level of long-chain unsaturated fats. Increasing this kind of unsaturated fat to normal decreases psychological symptoms.

Upper limit: the highest dose used in human research was 3 grams per day (reference[82]). This was not a study about EPO for the purpose of improving menopausal symptoms.

Side effects:

- Upset stomach
- Nausea
- Diarrhea
- Headache

How to Combine Supplements

You might have looked through this list of supplements, seen which one appeals to you, and started taking it. But then, you might have had a thought: "If supplement X decreases menopausal symptoms by __%, supplement Y decreases menopausal symptoms by __%, and supplement Z decreases menopausal symptoms by __%, I'll just take them all at the same time."

Don't do that.

Usually these **supplements are studied in isolation, and how your body would react if you were to take two or more at the same time is unknown**. They might have beneficial effects (that's what you're hoping for). But they might just cancel each other out.

To intelligently combine supplements, follow these steps:

<u>Step 1:</u> pick a supplement that you want to try.

Step 2: follow the steps from the section on *how to find the right supplement dose.*

Step 3: once you've found the right dose, stay there for 2-12 weeks, or until your symptoms change.

Step 4: add another supplement and repeat step 2.

With each new supplement you add, keep monitoring your menopausal symptoms, to see if that supplement works for you (if it improves your symptoms more than the supplement(s) that you're already taking) or if it negates the effects of the previous supplements.

It may be best to work with a medical professional who is knowledgeable when it comes to supplements, for the very important reason that supplements are rarely studied together, so little is known how they interact with each other when more than one is taken at a time.

Why Ineffective and Unproven Ingredients are Often Added to Supplements

So then, if most so-called "menopause supplements" either aren't effective at all, mostly ineffective, or unproven, why are they marketed as such? Is it all a complete lie, or is there even a shred of reason behind them? There are a few reasons why ineffective and/or unproven ingredients make it into menopause formulas:

1. Sometimes, **research done in mice or rats** shows that they help menopausal mice/rats reduce their symptoms. Too bad they aren't humans.

2. Some studies measure **short-term (as in, hours or days) changes in biochemical markers of estrogen, or certain neurotransmitters**. They then extrapolate to the long-term. But if the end result (menopausal symptoms) wasn't studied, that extrapolation is incorrect. There may be short-term changes in some biochemical markers, but nothing is said about menopausal symptoms.

3. In some studies, there's a mechanism by which symptoms could be reduced. That mechanism is plausible, but again, the end point of actual symptom reduction wasn't studied, so conclusions can't be made there.

4. Some studies are done in **petri dishes**. They don't study humans. They study an individual cell. A human is much more complex than that. Individual cells don't talk, and therefore, can't report symptoms.

5. **Dosages matter**. The studies showing effectiveness may use one dosage, whereas a supplement contains a much lower dosage than what's proven to be clinically effective.

6. **Amount of improvement matters**. It would be correct to say, "This supplement was shown to help people improve their symptoms." The question really is "How much?" If the answer is "It helped people reduce their symptoms by 0.01%", it's not really all that exciting.

Supplement companies know that the average person won't take the time to research the ingredients. And in all likelihood, the sales rep at your local health food store hasn't done the research either (even if they are a legit nutritionist). So the supplement companies will often use ineffective or unproven ingredients because they're impressive to the consumer, and they make sales.

That's not every supplement company, as there are a few good ones out there that make legitimately great formulations.

If you want a list of trustworthy supplement companies, just visit www.Mastering-Menopause.com, and I'll email them to you.

Chapter 9

Improving Sleep During Menopause and Beyond

Lots of postmenopausal women report their sleep getting worse after menopause. Considering how much good sleep contributes to quality of life and overall health, it's one of the most fundamental things to improve if you're not sleeping as well as you'd like.

In this chapter, you'll learn a few different techniques to try to help you sleep better (besides magnesium and melatonin).

But first...

Before we dive into the different sleep techniques, you first have to rule out sleep apnea. Sleep apnea is a condition where you briefly stop breathing at night, and end up waking up potentially hundreds of times throughout the night. But the wakeups are so short that you have no recollection of waking up. You might have been in bed for 8 hours, but only slept for 5 or 6. No wonder you feel tired.

One study[44] estimated that before menopause, about 16.8% of the population has sleep apnea. It's estimated that after menopause, that number goes up to 23.2%.

So before you try this technique, go to your doctor to ask them to send you to a sleep lab to get tested for sleep apnea.

After you've been tested, try the following techniques (not necessarily at the same time).

Technique #1: Write Down Your Thoughts

Lots of people report difficulty getting to sleep. Why? Because they have lots of racing thoughts, worries, or just things that they need to do the following day. They're afraid that if they fall asleep, they'll forget them.

A solution to that is to simply write down your thoughts, worries, or to-dos on a paper next to your bed, or on your phone/computer before you head to sleep.

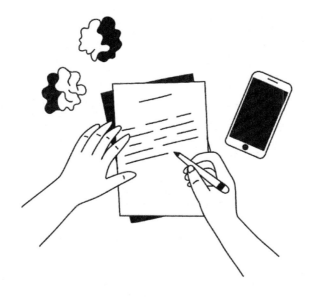

When it's not true insomnia, one study[40] showed that writing down your thoughts decreased the time it took to fall asleep after doing this for 3 days. With true insomnia, unfortunately, that technique doesn't seem to work. But stay tuned for later in this chapter, where I'll go over one of the strongest treatments for true insomnia.

Technique #2: Progressive Muscle Relaxation (PMR)

PMR is a very old technique, dating back to a psychologist from the 1920s named Dr. Edmund Jacobson. The purpose was to release unwanted and subconscious muscle tension. The theory was this would relieve the startle response common in anxiety and other conditions.

But does this work for poor sleep? At least one study[7] shows that it decreases the amount of time it takes to fall asleep (but not necessarily to stay asleep).

How do you do it?

<u>Step 1:</u> Tense your forehead muscles with 20% force for 6 seconds (this is obviously subjective. Just estimate what 20% of your maximal contraction would be).

<u>Step 2:</u> Relax the forehead. This is active relaxation. The goal is to relax the forehead as deeply as possible. The duration of relaxation should be 2-3 slow breaths.

<u>Step 3:</u> Tense the forehead with 40% force for 6 seconds.

<u>Step 4:</u> Repeat step 2

<u>Steps 5-onwards:</u> Keep tensing the forehead with higher and higher levels of force by 20%, until you reach 100%. Keep taking a 2-3 breath relaxation in between, while actively trying to deepen the relaxation.

Progressive Muscle Relaxation (PMR)

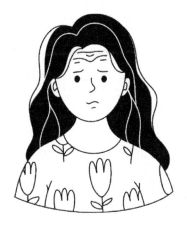 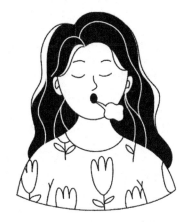

Repeat the same process with other muscles:

- Your eyes (shut them with varying levels of force).
- Your jaw.
- Your upper back/shoulders (just shrug – bring your shoulders towards your ears).
- Your mid-back.
- Your lower back.
- Your chest.
- Your abdominals.
- Your biceps.
- Your triceps.
- Your forearms.
- Your fingers (make a fist).
- Your buttocks.
- Your quads (front of the thighs).
- Your hamstrings (backs of your thighs).
- Your calves.

- Your feet.

All in all, this would take you about 45 minutes. If you want an abbreviated version, to do before sleep, just do your forehead, eyes, jaw, and upper back/shoulders.

PMR is typically not an exercise that you do forever, but for about 3-4 weeks. You should start to see results after about 3-10 days. So don't just do it once and conclude that it doesn't work. Give it a fair shot.

Technique #3: Cognitive-Behavioral Therapy for Insomnia (CBT-I)

Yes, there are sleep medications, there are supplements (melatonin, magnesium, etc.), and other home remedies (warm glass of milk, warm bath, etc.). But none of them are as tried-tested-and-true as CBT-I. Furthermore, **when you stop using them, the insomnia is back**. While they're good short-term solutions, they're not a long-term solution to insomnia. But CBT-I does have long-term effects.

One meta-analysis[18] found that CBT-I improved:

- Sleep efficiency (out of the total time in bed, how much was spent asleep).
- Sleep latency (how long it takes to fall asleep).
- How close to your intended wakeup time you wake up.

CBT-I is a **systematic way of reprogramming the thoughts and behaviours surrounding sleep**. Generally speaking, it's a 4–6-week program.

A key feature of CBT-I is something called "**sleep restriction therapy**." The goal is to associate the bed with sleep (as opposed to sleeplessness). The way it works is someone selects their wakeup time and works their way backwards from there.

Let's say that of their 8 hours in bed, they calculated that they're actually asleep for only 5 hours. So, in week 1, they'd only give themselves 5 hours of sleep. In other words, they would go to bed 5 hours before their desired wakeup time. The following week, maybe 5 hours and 15/30 minutes before their desired wakeup time, and it keeps on expanding by 15-30 minutes each week, until someone is sleeping a regular 7-9 hours per night.

There's quite a bit more to it than that, but that's the centrepiece.

CBT-I is about as close as there is to a **permanent solution to insomnia**, even if someone is elderly, even if their insomnia has been going on for decades, etc.

CBT-I can range from as much as $1500 (that's the highest I've seen), and as low as free (you can Google how to do it), and there are free apps that guide you. I don't want to mention any apps in this book, because apps come and go. I don't want to mention an app that no longer exists at the time you're reading this book).

If you want a great book on CBT-I, enter your email at www.Mastering-Menopause.com, and I'll send my recommendation to you.

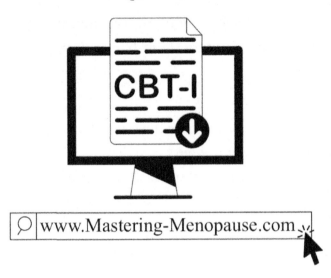

www.Mastering-Menopause.com

If you're wondering about exercise and nutrition as a tool for improving sleep: they enhance sleep in general, but do not help diagnosed insomnia. True insomnia is a lot more about ingrained behaviours and beliefs about sleep.

However, if you're having problems sleeping due to drops in hormone levels, well, the suggestions from the previous chapters on nutrition, exercise and supplements should help there as well.

Chapter 10

How Julie Lowered Her High Blood Pressure in a Month and Lost Weight at Age 59

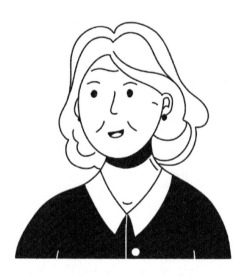

Meet Julie. She's a 59-year-old small business owner (her business is dog walking), and before she started working with us, she had **high blood pressure**, **a few pounds to lose**, **joint pain**, and was struggling with **menopausal symptoms**. Fast forward to now, and her blood pressure is normal, she fits into her old jeans again, she doesn't have any joint pain anymore, and her menopausal symptoms are gone.

How did she do it? That's exactly what we'll cover in this article.

You're going to learn:

- What Julie's life was like before her transformation.
- What Julie tried before to help her with her goals (and how it was working).
- The exercise strategies that she used to lower her blood pressure, get rid of joint pain and lose weight.
- The nutritional strategies that she used.
- The supplements we recommended.
- What results she achieved.
- The obstacles she faced along the way.
- How her life is different today.

And if you want to hear Julie tell her own story, she has recorded a video, which is available as an additional resource at www.Mastering-Menopause.com.

Julie's Life Before

Julie's been quite **active her whole life**. In her 30s, she played softball and badminton. In her 40s, she ran a few 5Ks and 10Ks. But fast-forward to menopause, and she gained a bunch of weight. Not a whole lot, but more than she wanted. Enough to **not fit into her favourite jeans** and clothes. Along with that, **her blood pressure went up** (it was around 140/90 mmHg on average), her joints (knees and lower back) started to hurt, and despite being in late menopause, she was still feeling the symptoms (night sweats, fatigue, and mood changes).

As a result, she was feeling – in her words – **crabby and cranky**, which was affecting the people around her (her family).

Factor in the back pain; between that and her mood, she **didn't feel like going out much with her friends and being social**.

What Julie Has Tried Before

Because Julie wasn't happy with how her body was doing, she's tried a bunch of things, like:

- **Calorie counting**. But as she'll admit – she likes beer. So she'd be in a caloric deficit, get hungry, binge, forget the deficit, and her weight would always go back up. No bueno.
- She has a dog walking business, so **she walks 10,000 steps per day 6-7 days per week**, no matter what – rain, shine, heat, cold, ice, etc. But despite that, she still couldn't fit into her old clothes, her blood pressure was high, and her knees and back hurt.

She didn't want to go on medications for either her blood pressure, weight (Ozempic), menopause or joint pain, and despite being active her whole life, she's **never stepped foot inside a gym before**.

But what she was doing obviously wasn't working, so she decided to do something she's never done before – hire a personal trainer.

Julie's Exercise Strategies

Weight loss is a lengthy process (generally 1 pound per week, if there's good compliance). Blood pressure normalization is a fast process (one British lady who read my blood pressure book commented on Amazon that her blood pressure went from "emergency high" to normal in a matter of 1 week of following the advice in the book). So at first, the program that Steven created for Julie was **oriented towards blood pressure reduction.**

It worked great. **In a matter of one month, her blood pressure went from an average of 140/90 mmHg to 120/80 mmHg.** Mission accomplished. And they were now free to work on the fat loss.

There's a specific way to exercise for blood pressure reduction, which is different from bone density, which is still different from diabetes, etc.

So Steven had Julie follow the blood pressure reduction exercise guidelines that we use with our clients, that are detailed in my book *High Blood Pressure Reversal.*

Here are just a few of the highlights of Julie's exercise routines and the thought process behind them:

- For the strength training portion, some of the exercise used were hip thrusts, lat pulldowns, incline pushups, cable rows and others.
- She was strength training twice per week and doing cardio 3 times per week.
- For cardio, the machine wasn't important, so whether she wanted to use the treadmill, elliptical, bike, swim, etc. didn't

matter. What mattered was the duration and the pulse. Her minimum pulse target was 122 beats per minute, and her prescribed duration was 30-50 minutes.

Again, the rationale behind all this is outlined in a special report that I've included at www.Mastering-Menopause.com.

There was a lot more to it than that, but these are the highlights of her program.

However if you just read about the exercises, you'd miss the "**secret sauce**" of the exercise program – the progression model, and the **workout-by-workout adjustments** that were made based on Julie's progress from the previous workout, energy/fatigue levels, injuries, and more. After all, **no exercise program should be a static program**, where you're doing the same exercises for the same weights, sets and reps every single time. **An exercise program should be dynamic, intelligently, purposefully, and systematically changing the exercise variables workout-by-workout** to move the person forward... as opposed to haphazardly changing the program whenever you feel like it, without rhyme or reason.

Julie's Nutritional Recommendations

At first, Julie's nutritional recommendations were oriented towards blood pressure reduction. The cool thing about **high blood pressure is that you can normalize it without weight loss**. So

Steven's recommendations at first were to have one of the following foods with each meal:

- Watermelon
- Melon
- Cucumber
- Celery
- Beets
- Garlic
- Spinach
- Sardines
- Dates
- Sun-dried tomatoes
- Dark chocolate
- Brazil nuts

Why these specific foods? Because there's more than one way to lower blood pressure. You can **increase potassium** (so some of these foods are specifically high potassium foods, like dates and sun-dried tomatoes), you can **increase magnesium** (some of these foods are specifically high magnesium foods, like dark chocolate and Brazil nuts), you can **increase omega 3s** (sardines and salmon are examples of high omega-3 foods), you can **use diuretics** (foods like watermelon, cucumbers and celery fit that bill). Or, you can make someone smell so bad that annoying people don't want to be around them, lowering blood pressure that way... hence the garlic recommendation 😉

Basically, each of the foods in this list was selected because it lowers high blood pressure by one or more different mechanisms.

After Julie's blood pressure normalized, it was time to turn their attention to her body fat. There are a million ways to lose body fat, and we've used different strategies with different clients. After all, as I always say, **nutrition must not only fit a person's body, but also their personality**.

Anyways, the overall message is that there's more than one way to get the job done.

Since Julie wasn't opposed to counting calories, that's what Steven had her do for the first 6 weeks, just to develop an awareness of how many calories she was eating. After that, he had her do a modest caloric reduction of 400 calories, and after 6 weeks, she dropped the calorie counting, and started more **intuitive eating**. Which worked for her – wait until you see the results later in this chapter.

However, Julie's goal wasn't weight loss. You can lose weight by losing muscle. You can also lose weight by losing bone. Neither one of those is desirable. So Julie's goal was **fat loss**. And the 2 keys to losing predominantly fat when you're in a caloric deficit are:

1. Adequate protein
2. Strength training

The strength training, you already know about. As for the protein, Steven calculated Julie's protein requirements, and together, they figured out which foods that she actually likes that would get her to her requirements.

Julie's Supplements

For Julie's high blood pressure, Steven recommended **magnesium glycinate** – one of the most common, and proven recommendations for high blood pressure.

Julie also had **osteopenia** (a stage before osteoporosis), so Steven recommended Type 1 collagen or collagen peptides. That's one of our most recommended bone health supplements, and the one that I recommend in my book, *Osteoporosis Reversal Secrets.*

Julie's Results

And now, it's the time we've all been waiting for – Julie's results. They're nothing short of impressive!

- As you know, her **blood pressure basically normalized in about 1 month** (from an average of 140/90 to 120/80).
- She **lost 9 pounds** of scale weight. But really, when you lose fat and gain muscle, what really happened is she likely lost about 14-15 pounds of fat and gained 5-6 pounds of muscle.
- She **lost 5.5 cm (about 2.25 inches) off her waist.**
- She **lost 30% of her belly fat** (from a skinfold of 37 mm to 26 mm)
- She **lost 29% of her love handle fat** (from a skinfold of 28 mm to 20 mm)

- Her leg and hip strength improved tremendously. Her hip thrusts went from 53 pounds, up to 163 pounds. That's a reflection of her **butt strength**.
- Her **upper body pushing strength more than doubled** – from a bench press of 28 pounds up to 58 pounds.
- Her **upper body pulling strength increased by 60%** - from a lat pulldown of 50 pounds up to 80 pounds.

And these are just the highlights. She had a lot more improvements in other areas as well.

Julie's Obstacles

We wish success was a straight line, but realistically, I tell my clients that **progress is like the stock market in a good year**. For the most part it goes up, but there's the occasional blip downwards.

In Julie's case, she **didn't see much weight loss for the first 4-5 weeks**. She saw fat loss, but her weight was staying the same. And although she intellectually knew this was going to happen, she had spent decades putting emotional energy into the number on the scale. It was a bit discouraging to not see that number move, at first.

However, that was somewhat by design. If you'll remember, we wanted to get the "easy stuff" done first – blood pressure normalization. So blood pressure normalization was the priority first, before fat loss. High blood pressure is a higher risk to a person's health than a few vanity pounds. She wasn't morbidly obese, so we tackled the bigger risk first. Once that risk was reduced, we set our sights on her weight and body fat.

And once we did, her weight started to drop nicely.

How Julie's Life is Different Now

Now that Julie is leaner, stronger and healthier, how is her life different today? Quite dramatically. The effects aren't just physical. They're **social**.

Before, because of Julie's back pain and not-so-great mood, she didn't want to go out with her friends. Now, she's up for it, because she doesn't have back pain anymore, and her mood is better.

Speaking of her friends, she's **getting lots of compliments on both her weight loss, but also how strong she looks**. After all, when she lost weight in the past, she didn't look good – because the focus was weight loss, and not fat loss. So she did it the wrong way – no strength training, and not enough protein. Now that she did it the right way, she's not just skinny – **she's lean**.

And along with that, **when she tries on her old jeans, they fit her great now**.

Overall, we're very proud of Julie, her work ethic, and how much progress she's made.

Chapter 11

How Stellis Lost 6 Inches Off Her Waist, At Age 83

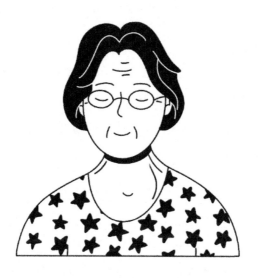

Meet Stellis. She's a retired administrator for the University of Toronto. She had a great life in retirement: an active life with her family and friends, volunteering for lots of activities with her church, travelling. But she felt she could do even better.

She felt like her life would be even better and more enjoyable if she lost weight, decreased her knee pain, and improved her strength and mobility. Fast forward a few months, and she lost 11 pounds and 6 inches off her waist, while getting into smaller dress sizes, and getting significantly stronger.

In this article, we'll cover:

- What Stellis has tried in the past to help her lose weight.
- What we learned about Stellis during our initial assessment.
- The exercise strategies that we used with Stellis.
- The nutritional strategies that we used with Stellis.
- The results we achieved.
- How her life is different now that she's 11 pounds lighter, 6 inches slimmer in the waist, and much stronger.

If you'd like to see Stellis tell her own story, I've included her video at www.Mastering-Menopause.com.

What Stellis Has Tried in the Past to Help Her Lose Fat

Excess body fat has been a long struggle for Stellis. And she's tried a lot of things like:

- **Diets** (many diets, including Atkins and Bernstein). Those didn't work, at least not in the long term.
- Going out for **daily walks**. And although it was enjoyable, it wasn't moving the needle.
- **Weight loss support group** (TOPS: Take Off Pounds Sensibly). While it was nice having peer support, she wasn't losing body fat. Also, the focus is on weight – not fat, or health.

She was frustrated that all those efforts yielded no results, at least not the ones she was looking for.

Around 2014 or 2015, I did a presentation for her TOPS group, and it was very well received.

Fast forward a few years and she decided to contact me to get started.

So as we do with all our clients, we started her off with an initial assessment.

What We Learned About Stellis During Our Initial Assessment

When it comes to designing an exercise and nutrition program, in order to personalize it, we have to know a lot of things, like:

- Someone's goal.
- What they're currently doing.
- What they've done in the past.
- Injuries.
- Medical conditions.
- Medications.
- Supplements.

...and other details.

In Stellis's case, she was already going for daily walks for an hour with a friend. In addition to that:

- She had high blood pressure.
- She had knee pain from arthritis.
- Other than that, she was pretty asymptomatic.

The Exercise Strategies That We Used

In terms of Stellis's program, here's what it looked like:

2 sets of 15-20 reps of:

- One-legged deadlifts
- Lat pulldowns
- Overhead press

Assisted squats or wall sits, depending on how her knees are feeling on any given day

- Seated rows
- Incline pushups
- Hamstring curls

Some rehabilitation exercises for her knees.

To look at this program alone, would really not do it justice. After all, the actual exercises are only the 4th most important variable in an exercise program. The top variable is the **progression model**, which is really the secret behind her success. If you want to know the second and third most important variables, I've included a special report about the most important factor in an exercise program at www.Mastering-Menopause.com.

The Nutritional Strategies Stellis Used

With every fat loss client, we try to identify whether their problem is **really nutritional, or whether it's more emotional,**

behavioral and logistical. About 5% of the time, it's nutritional. The rest of the time, emotional, behavioral and logistical.

Our approach to nutrition is not giving a massive overhaul. That would be called a "diet." Stellis has done diets in the past, and they haven't worked for her in the long term. So **why would we give her another diet, and just call it something different** (a "meal plan")?

As I talk about in chapter 4, you're much more likely to make long-term behavior change if you **focus on one skill at a time**. Thankfully, there are a million ways to reach the same goal, and different people can take different paths to get there.

The key is finding the **path of least resistance**. Because if you try to do something difficult, where you're likely to fail, you're much less likely to try again. But if you experience a small success, it'll reinforce that behavior, and you'll want to do more of it.

So after asking some diagnostic questions, we figured out that the most effective, but also easiest, least time consuming and tastiest way for Stellis to start long-term weight loss was by increasing her protein.

And that's all she did. We didn't make any other changes. We didn't ask her to eat more veggies, or use certain supplements, or anything else. That's the only thing we asked her to do.

And as we do with every client, we **took her body fat measurements every 2 weeks**. Sure enough, after 2 weeks of increasing her protein intake, she lost body fat. If it's working, keep going. So we kept on going without any changes. Another 2 weeks later, she lost even more body fat. So, we didn't make any changes, and kept on going. And on and on it went, until for 3 measurements in a row, she didn't make any progress.

The next step was to get her to **stop eating when she feels 80% full**, instead of 100% full. And again, we measured her 2 weeks later. She lost body fat from that. And another measurement 2 weeks later. More fat lost.

And those were basically the only 2 strategies Stellis needed to lose 11 pounds of fat, and drop 6 inches off her waist: more protein, and stop eating when she's 80% full.

When it comes to nutrition, very often, **simplicity works better than complexity**. But it takes **asking great questions**, and occasionally, experimentation to figure out what strategies to use for which person.

These 2 strategies worked great for Stellis, based on her preferences, schedule, personality, etc. They may not work for you. For you, other strategies may work. It just takes asking great questions to figure out which 1-3 strategies you need to implement. We're looking for **the one domino that knocks over other dominoes**.

The Results We Achieved

Theory and methods are nice, but there's a reason clients come to us: the bottom line. Can we help them reach their goals?

And I have to say, with Stellis, it's a resounding yes!

Since we meticulously measure and track our clients' progress, here are some highlights of Stellis's measurements:

- She lost 11 pounds: from 173, down to 162.
- She lost 6 inches off her waist: from 42.7 to 36.7.
- She added 30 pounds to her 1-legged deadlifts.
- Her upper body pulling strength improved by 20% (her lat pulldowns went from 50 pounds to 60).
- Her upper body pushing strength improved by 54% (her overhead press went from 18.5 pounds up to 28.5).
- Her recovery is better. It used to take her as much as 8 minutes to recover in between sets. Now it takes her about 3-4 minutes.

How Her Life is Different Now

Objective measurements are nice, but they're really just a proxy for us professionals to know whether we're on the right track or not. What really matters to our clients isn't so much their "gym numbers", but **how do exercise and nutrition enrich their life outside the gym**?

And turns out that for Stellis, her life has really improved:

- A lot of the clothes that she used to wear 11 pounds ago, she can no longer wear – they're too baggy now.
- She goes for daily walks with a friend of hers, who's much younger. Stellis used to have a hard time keeping up with her. Now, it's not a problem.

- **It's easier for her to get off the floor**. An underrated skill, but definitely on the minds of folks over 80 (and she's 83 now).
- She actually enjoys exercise now.
- It's easier for her to play with her grandkids.

So overall we're very proud of Stellis, and how far she's come in less than a year of exercise.

Chapter 12

Conclusion

You made it! You finished this book. Or maybe you just flipped to this chapter because you don't want the science. You just want the bottom line – "What do I do to improve my menopause symptoms, lose fat, get more toned, and have more energy?"

That's what you'll get in this section.

The Menopause Diet: What to Eat

- Health priorities during and after menopause:
  - Body fat
  - Menopausal symptoms
  - Fracture risk/bone density
  - Maintaining muscle strength (and function) into older age
  - Heart health
- How many calories should you eat:

Current bodyweight (in pounds) x 15 + calories spent on exercise – 10%.

  - Test body fat (not just weight) in 2 weeks. If the calorie deficit worked, keep it. If it didn't work, lower it by another 10%.
- Nutrition tracking apps have terrible accuracy. Instead, follow these steps:

o Write down what you ate.

o Write down how much of it you ate.

o Look up the nutritional value in a nutrition database (either one that you look up or the one provided for you at www.Mastering-Menopause.com) and multiply the calories by the serving size.

- Foods that reduce menopausal symptoms:
  o Flax seeds (2 tablespoons per day)
  o Soy and tofu (1 cup per day)
  o Beer (yes, really. Regular beer: 330 ml/day. Non-alcoholic beer: 660 ml/day)

- Calcium does not reduce fracture risk, but adequate protein does.

- Protein also helps with muscle mass and toning. How much protein should you get?

Activity Level	Under 60	Over 60
Sedentary	0.8-1.2 grams/kg/day	1.2-1.8 grams/kg/day
Cardio only	1.2-1.4 grams/kg/day	1.8-2.1 grams/kg/day
Strength training only	1.6-1.8 grams/kg/day	2.4-2.7 grams/kg/day
Cardio + strength training	1.6-1.8 grams/kg/day	2.4-2.7 grams/kg/day

- To maintain good heart health (as opposed to reversing existing heart problems):
    - Eat the right number of calories.
    - Make sure most of those calories are single-ingredient foods. For instance, how many ingredients are in a tomato? Just 1: tomato. How many ingredients are in chicken? Just 1: chicken. How many ingredients are in ice cream? More than 1.

End Emotional Eating

- Four most common reasons diets fail:
    - Emotional eating,
    - Stress eating,
    - Lack of planning,
    - Cravings.
- Techniques to address emotional eating:
    - Before you sit down to eat, rate your hunger and fullness on a -10 to +10 scale (between -10 and -1 means you're hungry; between +1 and +10 means you're full). If you score yourself higher than 0, wait until you drop below 0 to have a meal.
    - Name the emotion you're feeling at the time you're about to eat.
    - When you're eating, just eat – don't watch TV, scroll through your phone, work, or read the newspaper.
    - When you wake up in the morning, take 30 seconds to write down what you plan to eat later

that day, even if it's not the healthiest. You want it to be part of the plan.

- Design your environment to make it more conducive to healthy eating:
    - o Keep foods/drinks that aren't conducive to your health/fitness either out of the home, hidden by someone you live with, or out of plain sight.
    - o Keep foods that you want to eat more of (and drinks that you want to drink) in plain sight, and within arm's reach (e.g. vegetables, fruits, water and tea).
- Find a non-food reward that reinforces good behaviour. A good reward meets 4 criteria:
    - o Free.
    - o Takes less than 1 minute.
    - o Feels good.
    - o You can do immediately after the desired behaviour.
- If your plan to reduce emotional eating fails, analyze why it failed, and think about how you can prevent that the next time you're in the same situation.

Exercise for Menopause

- There are almost no differences between premenopausal and postmenopausal women in terms of their response to strength training, or how they should do it. They can gain very similar amount of both muscle and strength.

- There is a difference between premenopausal and postmenopausal women when it comes to cardio. Postmenopausal women need higher intensity (over 85% of the maximal heart rate).

Strength Training Exercise Prescription for Fat Loss

- **Frequency**: 2-3 days per week.
- **Intensity**: use a weight that gets you close to muscular failure (the point at which you can't do any more repetitions).
- **Volume**: 2-3 sets of 15-20 repetitions.
- **Full body workouts** (the actual exercises are coming up).
- **Circuit sets or supersets**.

Strength Training Exercise Prescription to Gain Strength Without Muscle Mass

- **Frequency**: 2-4 days per week.
- **Intensity**: use a weight that keeps you 3-4 repetitions from muscular failure.
- **Volume**: 3-5 sets of 3-5 repetitions.
- **Full body workouts** (the actual exercises are coming up).
- **Circuit sets, supersets or straight sets**. They all work for this purpose.

Strength Training Exercise Prescription to Gain Both Muscle Mass and Strength

- **Frequency**: 2-4 days per week.
- **Intensity**: use a weight that keeps you 0-2 repetitions from muscular failure.
- **Number of sets per muscle, per week**: 8-10. So if you're strength training twice per week, you'd be doing 4-5 sets per muscle per workout. If you're strength training three times per week, you'd be doing about 3 sets per muscle, per workout. If you're strength training four times per week, you'd be doing 2-3 sets per muscle, per workout.
- **Number of repetitions**: anywhere from 5-20. As long as you're **coming very close to muscular failure**.
- **Full body workouts** (the actual exercises are coming up).
- **Circuit sets, supersets or straight sets**.

Exercises:

- One-legged deadlifts
- Lat pulldowns
- Barbell overhead press
- Squats
- Seated rows
- Incline pushups
- Calf raises

Cardio Sample Program

Day 1

- **Interval duration**: 60 seconds
- **Intensity**: 85-90% of your HRmax
- **Number of intervals**: 4-12
- **When to start the next interval**: when your pulse comes down to 65% of your HRmax

Day 2

- **Interval duration:** 30 seconds
- **Intensity:** 85-90% of your HRmax
- **Number of intervals:** 6-18
- **When to start the next interval:** when your pulse comes down to 65% of your HRmax

Day 3

- **Interval duration:** 15 seconds
- **Intensity:** 90-95% of your top speed
- **Number of intervals:** 8-30
- **When to start the next interval:** when your pulse comes down to 65% of your HRmax

How to Reduce Muscular Aches and Pains During and After Menopause

- Lower estrogen levels increase damage to tendons and ligaments, and slow down recovery.
- Progesterone does not appear to affect tendons.
- Very little research exists on how testosterone affects tendons, but it's plausible that it has a strong effect.

Testosterone levels do decline during menopause, but not nearly as much as estrogen.

- What to do:
    - Get adequate protein.
    - Strength training, using the recommendations from the previous section.
    - Collagen supplementation. Specific collagen peptides, 5 grams/day.

Supplements for Menopause

Supplements that Work in Reducing Menopausal Symptoms:

- Black cohosh (up to 127 mg/day)
- Soy isoflavones (up to 100 mg/day)
- Sage leaf (AKA salvia officinalis): up to 100 mg, 3 times per day
- Red clover (up to 80 mg/day)

Ineffective Supplements for Menopausal Symptom Reduction:

- Dong quay (AKA angelica sinensis)
- Chaste tree berry (AKA vitex)

Unproven Supplements:

- Gamma oryzanol
- Hesperidin
- Inositol

- Multivitamins
- Fish oil
- Hop extract
- Evening primrose oil (AKA oenothera biennis)

How to Improve Sleep During and After Menopause

- First, get tested for sleep apnea in a sleep lab.
- Technique #1: write down your thoughts before you go to bed.
- Technique #2: progressive muscle relaxation (PMR)
  - o Contract and relax muscles with varying levels of force (20%, 40%, 60%, 80% and 100%).
  - o Contractions should be 6 seconds.
  - o Relaxations should be 2-3 breaths.
  - o During the relaxation phases, you should try to actively deepen the relaxation. Don't passively relax.
- Technique #3: cognitive-behavioural therapy for insomnia (CBT-I)
  - o Main feature: sleep restriction therapy
  - o Get a 1-week baseline of your sleep quality and quantity.
  - o Decide on your desired wake-up time.
  - o For 1 week, restrict your time in bed to only your total sleeping time (if you found that you spend 8 hours in bed, but only 5 hours asleep, go to bed 5 hours before your desired wake-up time).

o Each week, add 15-30 minutes to your bedtime.

Additional Resources at www.Mastering-Menopause.com:

- Special report: the pros and cons of different methods of testing body fat.
- Video explaining the different thyroid tests.
- A list of 49 different blood tests that you can ask your doctor for.
- First chapter of the book *Type 2 Diabetes Reversal Secrets.*
- First chapter of the book *High Blood Pressure Reversal Secrets.*
- First chapter of the book *Osteoporosis Reversal Secrets.*
- Nutrition database.
- Protein calculator.
- Additional resources on habit change.
- Videos of exercise demonstrations.
- Menopause symptom inventory.
- List of trusted supplement companies.
- Book recommendation on cognitive-behavioural therapy for insomnia (CBT-I).
- Special report: the most important factor in an exercise program.

Bibliography

1. Abd El-Kader, S. M., & Al-Jiffri, O. H. (2019). Impact of aerobic versus resisted exercise training on systemic inflammation biomarkers and quality of Life among obese post-menopausal women. *African health sciences*, *19*(4), 2881–2891. https://doi.org/10.4314/ahs.v19i4.10

2. Ahtiainen, J. P., Walker, S., Peltonen, H., Holviala, J., Sillanpää, E., Karavirta, L., Sallinen, J., Mikkola, J., Valkeinen, H., Mero, A., Hulmi, J. J., & Häkkinen, K. (2016). Heterogeneity in resistance training-induced muscle strength and mass responses in men and women of different ages. *AGE*, *38*(1). https://doi.org/10.1007/s11357-015-9870-1

3. Alati, R., Dunn, N., Purdie, D. M., Roche, A. M., Dennerstein, L., Darlington, S. J., Guthrie, J. R., & Green, A. C. (2007). Moderate alcohol consumption contributes to women's well-being through the menopausal transition. *Climacteric*, *10*(6), 491–499. https://doi.org/10.1080/13697130701739118

4. Almahmoud, Q. F., Alhaidar, S. M., Alkhenizan, A. H., Basudan, L. K., & Shafiq, M. (2023). Association Between Lipid Profile Measurements and Mortality Outcomes Among Older Adults in a Primary Care Setting: A Retrospective Cohort Study. *Curcus*, *15*(2), e35087. https://doi.org/10.7759/cureus.35087

5. A.O, O., C.J, U., S.C, M., & B.O, O. (2016). Between Estradiol and Thyroid Hormones in Menopausal Women. *IDOSR JOURNAL OF BIOCHEMISTRY, BIOTECHNOLOGY AND ALLIED FIELDS.* https://doi.org/https://www.idosr.org/wp-content/uploads/2017/08/IDOSR-JBBAF-11-2016-1-8.pdf

6. Baum, J. I., Kim, I. Y., & Wolfe, R. R. (2016). Protein Consumption and the Elderly: What Is the Optimal Level of Intake?. *Nutrients, 8*(6), 359. https://doi.org/10.3390/nu8060359

7. Bogdan, Vasile & Balazsi, Robert & Lupu, Viorel & Bogdan, Alexandru. (2009). Treating primary insomnia: A comparative study of self-help methods and progressive muscle relaxation. Journal of Cognitive and Behavioral Psychotherapies. 9. 67-82.

8. Bolla, K. N., & Sri.K.V , S. (2016). Effect of Soy Bean Consumption on Quality of Life of Middle Aged Women . *Advances in Life Science and Technology, 45.*

9. Brown TJ. Health benefits of weight reduction in postmenopausal women: a systematic review. British Menopause Society Journal. 2006;12(4):164-171. doi:10.1258/136218006779160599

10. Bzikowska-Jura, A., Sobieraj, P., & Raciborski, F. (2021). Low comparability of nutrition-related mobile apps against the Polish Reference Method—a validity study.

Nutrients,   *13*(8),   2868.
https://doi.org/10.3390/nu13082868

11. Cannon, J., Kay, D., Tarpenning, K. M., & Marino, F. E. (2007). Comparative effects of resistance training on peak isometric torque, muscle hypertrophy, voluntary activation and surface EMG between young and elderly women. *Clinical Physiology and Functional Imaging, 27*(2), 91–100.   https://doi.org/10.1111/j.1475-097x.2007.00719.x

12. Carpenter, C. L., Yan, E., Chen, S., Hong, K., Arechiga, A., Kim, W. S., Deng, M., Li, Z., & Heber, D. (2013). Body fat and body-mass index among a multiethnic sample of college-age men and women. *Journal of obesity, 2013,* 790654. https://doi.org/10.1155/2013/790654

13. Castelo-Branco, C., Gambacciani, M., Cano, A., Minkin, M. J., Rachoń, D., Ruan, X., Beer, A. M., Schnitker, J., Henneicke-von Zepelin, H. H., & Pickartz, S. (2021). Review & meta-analysis: isopropanolic black cohosh extract iCR for menopausal symptoms - an update on the evidence. *Climacteric : the journal of the International Menopause*   *Society, 24*(2),   109–119. https://doi.org/10.1080/13697137.2020.1820477

14. Chan, S., Gomes, A., & Singh, R. S. (2020). Is menopause still evolving? Evidence from a longitudinal study of multiethnic populations and its relevance to women's health. *BMC*   *women's*   *health, 20*(1),   74. https://doi.org/10.1186/s12905-020-00932-8

15. Charette, S. L., McEvoy, L., Pyka, G., Snow-Harter, C., Guido, D., Wiswell, R. A., & Marcus, R. (1991). Muscle hypertrophy response to resistance training in older women. *Journal of applied physiology (Bethesda, Md. : 1985), 70*(5),   1912–1916. https://doi.org/10.1152/jappl.1991.70.5.1912

16. Chen, J., Berkman, W., Bardouh, M., Ng, C. Y. K., & Allman-Farinelli, M. (2019). The use of a food logging app in the naturalistic setting fails to provide accurate measurements of nutrients and poses usability challenges. *Nutrition, 57,*   208-216. 10.1016/j.nut.2018.05.003

17. Chidi-Ogbolu, N., & Baar, K. (2019). Effect of estrogen on musculoskeletal performance and injury risk. *Frontiers in Physiology,*   *9.* https://doi.org/10.3389/fphys.2018.01834

18. Christelle, K., Zulkfili, M. M., Noor, N. M., & Draman, N. (2020). The effects of evening-primrose oil on menopausal symptoms: A systematic review and meta-analysis of randomized controlled trials. *Current Women s Health Reviews, 16*(4),   265–276. https://doi.org/10.2174/15734048169992007021627 50

19. Clark, D., Tomas, F., Withers, R. T., Chandler, C., Brinkman, M., Phillips, J., Berry, M., Ballard, F. J., & Nestel, P. (1994). Energy metabolism in free-living, 'large-eating' and 'small-eating' women: studies using 2H2(18)O. *The*

British journal of nutrition, *72*(1), 21–31. https://doi.org/10.1079/bjn19940006

20. Clark, D. G., Tomas, F. M., Withers, R. T., Brinkman, M., Berry, M. N., Oliver, J. R., Owens, P. C., Butler, R. N., Ballard, F. J., & Nestel, P. J. (1995). Differences in substrate metabolism between self-perceived 'large-eating' and 'small-eating' women. *International journal of obesity and related metabolic disorders : journal of the International Association for the Study of Obesity*, *19*(4), 245–252.

21. Colli, M. C., Bracht, A., Soares, A. A., de Oliveira, A. L., Bôer, C. G., de Souza, C. G., & Peralta, R. M. (2012). Evaluation of the efficacy of flaxseed meal and flaxseed extract in reducing menopausal symptoms. *Journal of medicinal food*, *15*(9), 840–845. https://doi.org/10.1089/jmf.2011.0228

22. Cornelissen, V. A., Verheyden, B., Aubert, A. E., & Fagard, R. H. (2009). Effects of aerobic training intensity on resting, exercise and post-exercise blood pressure, heart rate and heart-rate variability. *Journal of Human Hypertension*, *24*(3), 175–182. https://doi.org/10.1038/jhh.2009.51

23. Corsonello, A., Montesanto, A., Berardelli, M., De Rango, F., Dato, S., Mari, V., Mazzei, B., Lattanzio, F., & Passarino, G. (2010). A cross-section analysis of FT3 age-related changes in a group of old and oldest-old subjects, including centenarians' relatives, shows that a down-regulated thyroid function has a familial component and

is related to longevity. *Age and ageing*, *39*(6), 723–727. https://doi.org/10.1093/ageing/afq116

24. Davis, S. R., & Wahlin-Jacobsen, S. (2015). Testosterone in women--the clinical significance. *The lancet. Diabetes & endocrinology*, *3*(12), 980–992. https://doi.org/10.1016/S2213-8587(15)00284-3

25. Dietz, B. M., Hajirahimkhan, A., Dunlap, T. L., & Bolton, J. L. (2016). Botanicals and Their Bioactive Phytochemicals for Women's Health. *Pharmacological reviews*, *68*(4), 1026–1073. https://doi.org/10.1124/pr.115.010843

26. Dong, M., Guo, F., Yang, J., Liu, S., Tao, Z., Fang, Y., Zhang, C., Li, J., & Li, G. (2013). Detrimental effects of endogenous oestrogens on primary acute myocardial infarction among postmenopausal women. *Netherlands Heart Journal*, *21*(4), 175–180. https://doi.org/10.1007/s12471-012-0323-5

27. Erfiandi, F., Madjid, T. H., Ritonga, M. N., Susanto, H., & Susiarno, H. (2018). Effects of tofu consumption on menopause symptoms and equol level [7-hydroxy-3-(4 hydroxyphenyl) chroman]. *Journal of SAFOMS*, *6*(2), 117-121. https://doi.org/10.5005/jp-journals-10032-1152

28. Falconi, A. M., Gold, E. B., & Janssen, I. (2016). Th longitudinal relation of stress during the menopaus transition to fibrinogen concentrations: results from th Study of Women's Health Across the Nation. *Menopaus (New York, N.Y.)*, *23*(5), 518–52 https://doi.org/10.1097/GME.0000000000000579

29. Faubion, S. S., Sood, R., Thielen, J. M., & Shuster, L. T. (2015). Caffeine and menopausal symptoms. *Menopause*, *22*(2), 155–158. https://doi.org/10.1097/gme.0000000000000301

30. Fujii, M., Butler, J. P., & Sasaki, H. (2018). Gamma-oryzanol for behavioural and psychological symptoms of dementia. *Psychogeriatrics : the official journal of the Japanese Psychogeriatric Society*, *18*(2), 151–152. https://doi.org/10.1111/psyg.12303

31. Ghazanfarpour, M., Sadeghi, R., Latifnejad Roudsari, R., Khadivzadeh, T., Khorsand, I., Afiat, M., & Esmaeilizadeh, M. (2016). Effects of flaxseed and Hypericum perforatum on hot flash, vaginal atrophy and estrogen-dependent cancers in menopausal women: a systematic review and meta-analysis. *Avicenna journal of phytomedicine*, *6*(3), 273–283.

32. Ghazanfarpour, M., Sadeghi, R., Roudsari, R. L., Khorsand, I., Khadivzadeh, T., & Muoio, B. (2016). Red clover for treatment of hot flashes and menopausal symptoms: A systematic review and meta-analysis. *Journal of obstetrics and gynaecology : the journal of the Institute of Obstetrics and Gynaecology*, *36*(3), 301–311. https://doi.org/10.3109/01443615.2015.1049249

33. Gholizadeh, S., Sadatmahalleh, S. J., & Ziaei, S. (2018). The association between estradiol levels and cognitive function in postmenopausal women. *International journal of reproductive biomedicine*, *16*(7), 455–458.

34. Giordano, D., Corrado, F., Santamaria, A., Quattrone, S., Pintaudi, B., Di Benedetto, A., & D'Anna, R. (2011). Effects of myo-inositol supplementation in postmenopausal women with metabolic syndrome: a perspective, randomized, placebo-controlled study. *Menopause (New York, N.Y.), 18*(1), 102–104. https://doi.org/10.1097/gme.0b013e3181e8e1b1

35. Gościniak, A., Szulc, P., Zielewicz, W., Walkowiak, J., & Cielecka-Piontek, J. (2023). Multidirectional Effects of Red Clover (*Trifolium pratense* L.) in Support of Menopause Therapy. *Molecules (Basel, Switzerland), 28*(13), 5178. https://doi.org/10.3390/molecules28135178

36. Gregorio, L., Brindisi, J., Kleppinger, A., Sullivan, R., Mangano, K. M., Bihuniak, J. D., Kenny, A. M., Kerstetter, J. E., & Insogna, K. L. (2014). Adequate dietary protein is associated with better physical performance among post-menopausal women 60-90 years. *The journal of nutrition, health & aging, 18*(2), 155–160. https://doi.org/10.1007/s12603-013-0391-2

37. Griffiths, C., Harnack, L., & Pereira, M. (2018). Assessment of the accuracy of nutrient calculations of five popular nutrition tracking applications. *Public Health Nutrition, 21*(8), 1495-1502. doi:10.1017/S1368980018000393

38. Hansen M. (2018). Female hormones: do they influence muscle and tendon protein metabolism?. *The Proceedings*

of the Nutrition Society, 77(1), 32–41. https://doi.org/10.1017/S0029665117001951

39. Hansen, M., Kongsgaard, M., Holm, L., Skovgaard, D., Magnusson, S. P., Qvortrup, K., Larsen, J. O., Aagaard, P., Dahl, M., Serup, A., Frystyk, J., Flyvbjerg, A., Langberg, H., & Kjaer, M. (2009). Effect of estrogen on tendon collagen synthesis, tendon structural characteristics, and biomechanical properties in postmenopausal women. *Journal of applied physiology (Bethesda, Md. : 1985), 106*(4), 1385–1393. https://doi.org/10.1152/japplphysiol.90935.2008

40. Harvey, A. G., & Farrell, C. (2003). The efficacy of a Pennebaker-like writing intervention for poor sleepers. *Behavioral sleep medicine, 1*(2), 115–124. https://doi.org/10.1207/S15402010BSM0102_4

41. Heath, C., & Heath, D. (2011). *Switch: How to change things when change is hard.* Broadway Books.

42. Heyerick, A., Vervarcke, S., Depypere, H., Bracke, M., & De Keukeleire, D. (2006). A first prospective, randomized, double-blind, placebo-controlled study on the use of a standardized hop extract to alleviate menopausal discomforts. *Maturitas, 54*(2), 164–175. https://doi.org/10.1016/j.maturitas.2005.10.005

43. Hirata, J. D., Swiersz, L. M., Zell, B., Small, R., & Ettinger, B. (1997). Does Dong Quai have estrogenic effects in postmenopausal women? A double-blind, placebo-

controlled trial. *Fertility and Sterility, 68*(6), 981–986. https://doi.org/10.1016/s0015-0282(97)00397-x

44. Hirotsu, C., Albuquerque, R. G., Nogueira, H., Hachul, H., Bittencourt, L., Tufik, S., & Andersen, M. L. (2017). The relationship between sleep apnea, metabolic dysfunction and inflammation: The gender influence. *Brain, Behavior, and Immunity, 59,* 211–218. https://doi.org/10.1016/j.bbi.2016.09.005

45. Holzmann SL, Pröll K, Hauner H, Holzapfel C (2017) Nutrition apps: quality and limitations. An explorative investigation on the basis of selected apps. Ernahrungs Umschau 64(5): 80–89

46. Jerger, S., Centner, C., Lauber, B., Seynnes, O., Sohnius, T., Jendricke, P., Oesser, S., Gollhofer, A., & König, D. (2022). Effects of specific collagen peptide supplementation combined with resistance training on Achilles tendon properties. *Scandinavian journal of medicine & science in sports, 32*(7), 1131–1141. https://doi.org/10.1111/sms.14164

47. Kadoglou, N. P. E., Biddulph, J. P., Rafnsson, S. B., Trivella, M., Nihoyannopoulos, P., & Demakakos, P. (2017). The association of ferritin with cardiovascular and all-cause mortality in community-dwellers: The English longitudinal study of ageing. *PloS one, 12*(6), e0178994. https://doi.org/10.1371/journal.pone.0178994

48. Kanis, J. A., Johansson, H., Oden, A., De Laet, C., Johnell, O., Eisman, J. A., McCloskey, E., Mellstrom, D., Pols, H., Reeve,

J., Silman, A., & Tenenhouse, A. (2004). A meta-analysis of milk intake and fracture risk: Low utility for case finding. *Osteoporosis International,* *16*(7), 799–804. https://doi.org/10.1007/s00198-004-1755-6

49. Kenda, M., Glavač, N. K., Nagy, M., Sollner Dolenc, M., & On Behalf Of The Oemonom (2021). Herbal Products Used in Menopause and for Gynecological Disorders. *Molecules (Basel, Switzerland),* *26*(24), 7421. https://doi.org/10.3390/molecules26247421

50. Khalafi, M., Malandish, A., & Rosenkranz, S. K. (2021). The impact of exercise training on inflammatory markers in postmenopausal women: A systemic review and meta analysis. *Experimental gerontology,* *150,* 111398. https://doi.org/10.1016/j.exger.2021.111398

51. Khalafi, M., Sakhaei, M. H., Habibi Maleki, A., Rosenkranz, S. K., Pourvaghar, M. J., Fang, Y., & Korivi, M. (2023). Influence of exercise type and duration on cardiorespiratory fitness and muscular strength in post-menopausal women: A systematic review and meta-analysis. *Frontiers in Cardiovascular Medicine,* *10.* https://doi.org/10.3389/fcvm.2023.1190187

52. Kretzschmar, J., Babbitt, D. M., Diaz, K. M., Feairheller, D. L., Sturgeon, K. M., Perkins, A. M., Veerabhadrappa, P., Williamson, S. T., Ling, C., Lee, H., Grimm, H., Thakkar, S. R., Crabbe, D. L., Kashem, M. A., & Brown, M. D. (2014). A standardized exercise intervention differentially affects premenopausal and postmenopausal African-American

women. *Menopause (New York, N.Y.)*, *21*(6), 579–584. https://doi.org/10.1097/GME.0000000000000133

53. Laakmann, E., Grajecki, D., Doege, K., zu Eulenburg, C., & Buhling, K. J. (2012). Efficacy of Cimicifuga racemosa, Hypericum perforatum and Agnus castus in the treatment of climacteric complaints: a systematic review. *Gynecological endocrinology : the official journal of the International Society of Gynecological Endocrinology*, *28*(9), 703–709. https://doi.org/10.3109/09513590.2011.650772

54. Lee, I. M., Djoussé, L., Sesso, H. D., Wang, L., & Buring, J. E. (2010). Physical activity and weight gain prevention. *JAMA*, *303*(12), 1173–1179. https://doi.org/10.1001/jama.2010.312

55. Lemieux, F. C., Filion, M. E., Barbat-Artigas, S., Karelis, A. D., & Aubertin-Leheudre, M. (2014). Relationship between different protein intake recommendations with muscle mass and muscle strength. *Climacteric : the journal of the International Menopause Society*, *17*(3), 294–300. https://doi.org/10.3109/13697137.2013.829440

56. Li, S., Hou, L., Zhu, S., Yi, Q., Liu, W., Zhao, Y., Wu, F., Li, X., Pan, A., & Song, P. (2022). Lipid Variability and Risk of Cardiovascular Diseases and All-Cause Mortality: Systematic Review and Meta-Analysis of Cohort Studies. *Nutrients*, *14*(12), 2450. https://doi.org/10.3390/nu14122450

57. Lindsay, R., Gallagher, J. C., Kleerekoper, M., & Pickar, J. H. (2002). Effect of lower doses of conjugated equine estrogens with and without medroxyprogesterone acetate on bone in early postmenopausal women. *JAMA, 287*(20), 2668–2676. https://doi.org/10.1001/jama.287.20.2668

58. Liske, E., Hänggi, W., Henneicke-von Zepelin, H. H., Boblitz, N., Wüstenberg, P., & Rahlfs, V. W. (2002). Physiological investigation of a unique extract of black cohosh (Cimicifugae racemosae rhizoma): a 6-month clinical study demonstrates no systemic estrogenic effect. *Journal of women's health & gender-based medicine, 11*(2), 163–174. https://doi.org/10.1089/152460902753645308

59. Lovering, R. M., & Romani, W. A. (2005). Effect of testosterone on the female anterior cruciate ligament. *American journal of physiology. Regulatory, integrative and comparative physiology, 289*(1), R15–R22. https://doi.org/10.1152/ajpregu.00829.2004

60. Malandish, A., & Rahmati-Yamchi, M. (2022). The effect of moderate intensity aerobic exercise on cardiovascular function, cardiorespiratory fitness and estrogen receptor alpha gene in overweight/obese postmenopausal women: A randomized controlled trial. *Journal of Molecular and Cellular Cardiology Plus, 2,* 100026. 10.1016/j.jmccpl.2022.100026

61. Mandrup, C. M., Egelund, J., Nyberg, M., Lundberg Slingsby, M. H., Andersen, C. B., Løgstrup, S., Bangsbo, J., Suetta, C., Stallknecht, B., & Hellsten, Y. (2017). Effects of high-intensity training on cardiovascular risk factors in premenopausal and postmenopausal women. *American Journal of Obstetrics and Gynecology, 216*(4), 384.e1-384.e11. 10.1016/j.ajog.2016.12.017

62. McTiernan, A., Tworoger, S. S., Ulrich, C. M., Yasui, Y., Irwin, M. L., Rajan, K. B., Sorensen, B., Rudolph, R. E., Bowen, D., Stanczyk, F. Z., Potter, J. D., & Schwartz, R. S. (2004). Effect of exercise on serum estrogens in postmenopausal women: a 12-month randomized clinical trial. *Cancer research, 64*(8), 2923–2928. https://doi.org/10.1158/0008-5472.can-03-3393

63. Messina M. (2016). Soy and Health Update: Evaluation of the Clinical and Epidemiologic Literature. *Nutrients, 8*(12), 754. https://doi.org/10.3390/nu8120754

64. Mistura, L., Comendador Azcarraga, F. J., D'Addezio, L., Martone, D., & Turrini, A. (2021). An Italian case study for assessing nutrient intake through nutrition-related mobile apps. *Nutrients, 13*(9), 3073. https://doi.org/10.3390/nu13093073

65. Monninkhof, E. M., Velthuis, M. J., Peeters, P. H., Twisk, J. W., & Schuit, A. J. (2009). Effect of exercise on postmenopausal sex hormone levels and role of body fat: a randomized controlled trial. *Journal of clinical oncology : official journal of the American Society of Clinica*

Oncology, 27(27),   4492–4499.
https://doi.org/10.1200/JCO.2008.19.7459

66. Myung, S., Ju, W., Choi, H., & Kim, S. (2009). Soy intake and risk of endocrine-related gynaecological cancer: A meta-analysis. *BJOG: An International Journal of Obstetrics & Gynaecology, 116*(13), 1697–1705. https://doi.org/10.1111/j.1471-0528.2009.02322.x

67. O'Sullivan, M., & Overton, C. (2016). Managing debilitating menopausal symptoms. *The Practitioner, 260*(1791), 17–3.

68. Perna, S., Peroni, G., Miccono, A., Riva, A., Morazzoni, P., Allegrini, P., Preda, S., Baldiraghi, V., Guido, D., & Rondanelli, M. (2016). Multidimensional Effects of Soy Isoflavone by Food or Supplements in Menopause Women: a Systematic Review and Bibliometric Analysis. *Natural product communications, 11*(11), 1733–1740.

69. Pimenta, F., Maroco, J., Ramos, C., & Leal, I. (2014). Predictors of weight variation and weight gain in peri- and post-menopausal women. *Journal of health psychology, 19*(8),   993–1002. https://doi.org/10.1177/1359105313483153

70. Pontzer, H., Yamada, Y., Sagayama, H., Ainslie, P. N., Andersen, L. F., Anderson, L. J., Arab, L., Baddou, I., Bedu-Addo, K., Blaak, E. E., Blanc, S., Bonomi, A. G., Bouten, C. V. C., Bovet, P., Buchowski, M. S., Butte, N. F., Camps, S. G., Close, G. L., Cooper, J. A., Cooper, R., ... IAEA DLW Database

Consortium (2021). Daily energy expenditure through the human life course. *Science (New York, N.Y.), 373*(6556), 808–812. https://doi.org/10.1126/science.abe5017

71. Proietto J. (2017). Obesity and weight management at menopause. *Australian family physician, 46*(6), 368–370.

72. Poehlman, E. T., Goran, M. I., Gardner, A. W., Ades, P. A., Arciero, P. J., Katzman-Rooks, S. M., Montgomery, S. M., Toth, M. J., & Sutherland, P. T. (1993). Determinants of decline in resting metabolic rate in aging females. *The American journal of physiology, 264*(3 Pt 1), E450–E455. https://doi.org/10.1152/ajpendo.1993.264.3.E450

73. Poehlman ET, Tchernof A. Traversing the menopause: changes in energy expenditure and body composition. Coronary Artery Disease. 1998 ;9(12):799-803. PMID: 9894924.

74. Praet, S. F. E., Purdam, C. R., Welvaert, M., Vlahovich, N., Lovell, G., Burke, L. M., Gaida, J. E., Manzanero, S., Hughes, D., & Waddington, G. (2019). Oral Supplementation of Specific Collagen Peptides Combined with Calf-Strengthening Exercises Enhances Function and Reduces Pain in Achilles Tendinopathy Patients. *Nutrients, 11*(1), 76. https://doi.org/10.3390/nu11010076

75. Reame, N. E., Lukacs, J. L., Padmanabhan, V., Eyvazzadeh, A. D., Smith, Y. R., & Zubieta, J. K. (2008). Black cohosh has central opioid activity in postmenopausal women: evidence from naloxone blockade and positron emission

tomography neuroimaging. *Menopause (New York, N.Y.), 15*(5), 832–840. https://doi.org/10.1097/gme.0b013e318169332a

76. Rolland, Y. M., Perry, H. M., 3rd, Patrick, P., Banks, W. A., & Morley, J. E. (2007). Loss of appendicular muscle mass and loss of muscle strength in young postmenopausal women. *The journals of gerontology. Series A, Biological sciences and medical sciences, 62*(3), 330–335. https://doi.org/10.1093/gerona/62.3.330

77. Saccomani, S., Lui-Filho, J. F., Juliato, C. R., Gabiatti, J. R., Pedro, A. O., & Costa-Paiva, L. (2017). Does obesity increase the risk of hot flashes among midlife women?: a population-based study. *Menopause (New York, N.Y.), 24*(9), 1065–1070. https://doi.org/10.1097/GME.0000000000000884

78. Sadahiro, R., Matsuoka, L. N., Zeng, B. S., Chen, K. H., Zeng, B. Y., Wang, H. Y., Chu, C. S., Stubbs, B., Su, K. P., Tu, Y. K., Wu, Y. C., Lin, P. Y., Chen, T. Y., Chen, Y. W., Suen, M. W., Hopwood, M., Yang, W. C., Sun, C. K., Cheng, Y. S., Shiue, Y. L., ... Tseng, P. T. (2023). Black cohosh extracts in women with menopausal symptoms: an updated pairwise meta-analysis. *Menopause (New York, N.Y.), 30*(7), 766–773. https://doi.org/10.1097/GME.0000000000002196

79. Safdari, F., Motaghi Dastenaei, B., Kheiri, S., & Karimiankakolaki, Z. (2021). Effect of Evening Primrose Oil on Postmenopausal Psychological Symptoms: A Triple-Blind Randomized Clinical Trial. *Journal of*

menopausal   medicine, *27*(2),   58–65.
https://doi.org/10.6118/jmm.21010

80. Schindler   A.   E.   (2003).   Thyroid   function   and
postmenopause. *Gynecological endocrinology : the official
journal of the International Society of Gynecological
Endocrinology, 17*(1), 79–85.

81. Sempos, C. T., Looker, A. C., Gillum, R. E., McGee, D. L.,
Vuong, C. V., & Johnson, C. L. (2000). Serum ferritin and
death from all causes and cardiovascular disease: the
NHANES II Mortality Study. National Health and Nutrition
Examination Study. *Annals of epidemiology, 10*(7), 441–
448. https://doi.org/10.1016/s1047-2797(00)00068-5

82. Sharma, N., Gupta, A., Jha, P. K., & Rajput, P. (2012).
Mastalgia   cured!   Randomized   trial   comparing
centchroman   to   evening   primrose   oil. *The breast
journal, 18*(5),   509–510.
https://doi.org/10.1111/j.1524-4741.2012.01288.x

83. Simpson, E. E. A., Furlong, O. N., Parr, H. J., Hodge, S. J
Slevin, M. M., McSorley, E. M., McCormack, J. M
McConville, C., & Magee, P. J. (2019). The effect of
randomized 12-week soy drink intervention on everyda
mood in postmenopausal women. *Menopause (New York
N.Y.), 26*(8),   867–87
https://doi.org/10.1097/GME.0000000000001322

84. Singh, P. N., Haddad, E., Knutsen, S. F., & Fraser, G.
(2001). The effect of menopause on the relation betwee
weight gain and mortality among women. *Menopau*

(New York, N.Y.), 8(5), 314–320.
https://doi.org/10.1097/00042192-200109000-00004

85. Sites, C. K., Toth, M. J., Cushman, M., L'Hommedieu, G. D., Tchernof, A., Tracy, R. P., & Poehlman, E. T. (2002). Menopause-related differences in inflammation markers and their relationship to body fat distribution and insulin-stimulated glucose disposal. *Fertility and sterility, 77*(1), 128–135. https://doi.org/10.1016/s0015-0282(01)02934-x

86. Sowers, M. R., Randolph, J. F., Zheng, H., Jannausch, M., McConnell, D., Kardia, S. R., Crandall, C. J., & Nan, B. (2011). Genetic polymorphisms and obesity influence estradiol decline during the menopause. *Clinical endocrinology, 74*(5), 618–623. https://doi.org/10.1111/j.1365-2265.2010.03968.x

87. Stijak, L., Kadija, M., Djulejić, V., Aksić, M., Petronijević, N., Marković, B., Radonjić, V., Bumbaširević, M., & Filipović, B. (2015). The influence of sex hormones on anterior cruciate ligament rupture: female study. *Knee surgery, sports traumatology, arthroscopy : official journal of the ESSKA, 23*(9), 2742–2749. https://doi.org/10.1007/s00167-014-3077-3

88. Thomas, E., Gentile, A., Lakicevic, N., Moro, T., Bellafiore, M., Paoli, A., Drid, P., Palma, A., & Bianco, A. (2021). The effect of resistance training programs on lean body mass in postmenopausal and elderly women: a meta-analysis of observational studies. *Aging clinical and experimental*

research, 33(11),   2941–2952.
https://doi.org/10.1007/s40520-021-01853-8

89. Tosi, M., Radice, D., Carioni, G., Vecchiati, T., Fiori, F., Parpinel, M., & Gnagnarella, P. (2021). Accuracy of applications to monitor food intake: Evaluation by comparison with 3-d food diary. *Nutrition, 84,* 111018. 10.1016/j.nut.2020.111018

90. Trius-Soler, M., Marhuenda-Muñoz, M., Laveriano-Santos, E. P., Martínez-Huélamo, M., Sasot, G., Storniolo, C. E., Estruch, R., Lamuela-Raventós, R. M., & Tresserra-Rimbau, A. (2021). Moderate consumption of beer (with and without ethanol) and menopausal symptoms: Results from a parallel clinical trial in postmenopausal women. *Nutrients,* *13*(7), 2278. https://doi.org/10.3390/nu13072278

91. Wanders, J. O., Bakker, M. F., Veldhuis, W. B., Peeters, P. H., & van Gils, C. H. (2015). The effect of weight change on changes in breast density measures over menopause in a breast cancer screening cohort. *Breast cancer research : BCR, 17*(1), 74. https://doi.org/10.1186/s13058-015-0583-2

92. Wang, Q., Liu, X., & Ren, S. (2020). Tofu intake is inversely associated with risk of breast cancer: A meta-analysis of observational studies. *PLOS ONE, 15*(1). https://doi.org/10.1371/journal.pone.0226745

93. Wang, Y. Y., Yang, Y., Rao, W. W., Zhang, S. F., Zeng, L. N., Zheng, W., Ng, C. H., Ungvari, G. S., Zhang, L., & Xiang, Y. T.

(2020). Cognitive behavioural therapy monotherapy for insomnia: A meta-analysis of randomized controlled trials. *Asian journal of psychiatry, 49,* 101828. https://doi.org/10.1016/j.ajp.2019.10.008

94. Wilfried, D., Nina, C. D. G., & Silvia, B. (2021). Effectiveness of Menosan® *Salvia officinalis* in the treatment of a wide spectrum of menopausal complaints. A double-blind, randomized, placebo-controlled, clinical trial. *Heliyon, 7*(2), e05910. https://doi.org/10.1016/j.heliyon.2021.e05910

95. Woods, N. F., Carr, M. C., Tao, E. Y., Taylor, H. J., & Mitchell, E. S. (2006). Increased urinary cortisol levels during the menopausal transition. *Menopause (New York, N.Y.), 13*(2), 212–221. https://doi.org/10.1097/01.gme.0000198490.57242.2e

96. Woods, N. F., Mitchell, E. S., & Smith-Dijulio, K. (2009). Cortisol levels during the menopausal transition and early postmenopause: observations from the Seattle Midlife Women's Health Study. *Menopause (New York, N.Y.), 16*(4), 708–718. https://doi.org/10.1097/gme.0b013e318198d6b2

97. Tamara, J. B. (2006). Health benefits of weight reduction in postmenopausal women: a systematic review. *British Menopause Society Journal, 12*(4), 164-171. 10.1258/136218006779160599

98. Zacho, J., Tybjaerg-Hansen, A., & Nordestgaard, B. G. (2010). C-reactive protein and all-cause mortality--the

Copenhagen City Heart Study. *European heart journal, 31*(13), 1624–1632. https://doi.org/10.1093/eurheartj/ehq103

99. Zeidabadi, A., Yazdanpanahi, Z., Dabbaghmanesh, M. H., Sasani, M. R., Emamghoreishi, M., & Akbarzadeh, M. (2020). The effect of Salvia officinalis extract on symptoms of flushing, night sweat, sleep disorders, and score of forgetfulness in postmenopausal women. *Journal of family medicine and primary care, 9*(2), 1086–1092. https://doi.org/10.4103/jfmpc.jfmpc_913_19

Other Books by This Author

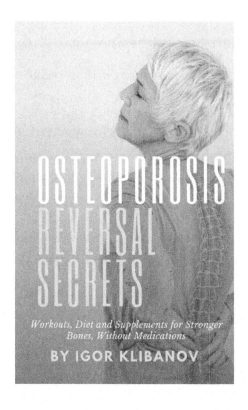

Osteoporosis Reversal Secrets: Workouts, Diet and upplements for Stronger Bones, Without Medications

If you have osteoporosis, you may be concerned about the onsequences, like falling, fracturing or breaking a bone, and having) be dependent on family for care. Fortunately, there are simple ʾays to reverse your osteoporosis <u>without</u> spending hours at the /m, cutting out the foods that you love, or taking dangerous edications. And there's more than 1 way to do it. If one doesn't ɔpeal to you, try a different method from this book.

In this book, you will learn:

- About the osteoporosis workout.

- Exercises for osteoporosis that reduce fracture risk by over 50%

- Osteoporosis supplements for women and men: 5 effective supplements, 1 ineffective supplement (even though it's included in almost every formula for bone), 11 unproven supplements.

- The 3 types of exercise that you have to do to minimize your fracture risk and have better bones

- A common nutrient frequently recommended for osteoporosis – that DOESN'T work

- The single most important nutrient for strong bones (hint it's not calcium or vitamin D)

...and so much more.

To get a copy of this book, visit **https://amzn.to/43xhgRD**.

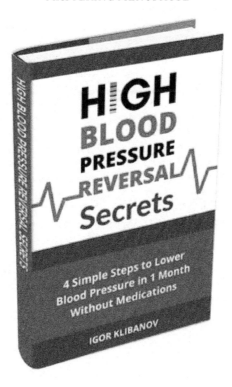

High Blood Pressure Reversal Secrets: 4 Simple Steps to Lower Blood Pressure in 1 Month Without Medications

If you have high blood pressure (AKA hypertension), you may be concerned about the consequences, like heart attacks, strokes, vision loss, and others.

Fortunately, there are simple ways that don't take a lot of time or effort that can reverse your high blood pressure, and there's more than 1 way to do it. If one method doesn't appeal to you, pick a different method.

In this book you will learn:

- Why you don't have to lose weight to lower your blood pressure
- A simple exercise for hypertension that you can do for 8 minutes per day, 3 days per week that can lower your blood pressure by 15.3/7.8 mmHg in just a few weeks
- A list of regular foods to add to your diet that will help you lower your blood pressure
- 3 proven supplements that can lower your blood pressure by more than 10/4 mmHg, and have no side effects
- Natural remedies for high blood pressure
- How 47-year-old George used our methods to reverse his high blood pressure in 12 weeks

...and so much more.

To get a copy of this book, visit **https://amzn.to/3wuGFKP**.

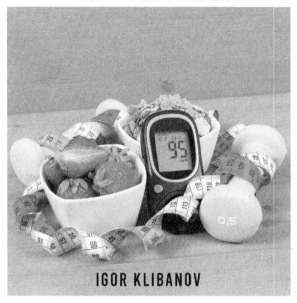

Type 2 Diabetes Reversal Secrets: 4 Simple Steps to Lower Blood Sugar in 1 Month, Without Medications

If you have type 2 diabetes, you may be concerned about the consequences, like vision loss, dry skin, heart attacks, strokes, and others. Fortunately, there are simple ways that don't take a lot of time or effort that can help with type 2 diabetes reversal, and there's more than 1 way to do it. If one method doesn't appeal to you, pick a different method.

In this diabetes book you will learn everything it takes when it comes to mastering diabetes, including:

- The difference between reversing diabetes and the diabetes cure (they're not the same)

- Diabetes and weight loss: why you don't need to lose weight to reverse your diabetes (but if you need to lose weight, following the advice in this book will still help)

- The 4 most important components of the diabetes eating plan AKA diabetes reversal diet (hint: carbs are only the 3rd most important factor)

- The ultimate diabetes food list: delicious and simple everyday foods that can lower or normalize high blood sugar levels

- Intermittent fasting for diabetes: does it work?

- How to reverse diabetes without drugs

- 4 effective diabetes supplements that can lower blood sugar levels (HbA1C) by at least 1.0%

- 5 ineffective supplements that still get included in blood sugar formulas

- 6 unproven supplements for diabetes

- The most effective exercise program for diabetes. Cardio or strength training? How many times per week? How long? How much?

- The mechanisms: how does exercise help diabetes?

- Why having a normal blood sugar level is not enough, and 4 OTHER tests you need to run to have a comprehensive picture of your diabetes (type 2)

- One common sleep condition that could be raising your insulin levels.

...and other diabetes essentials you need to know for proper diabetes management.

If you want to pick up a copy, go to https://amzn.to/3DaBqmR.

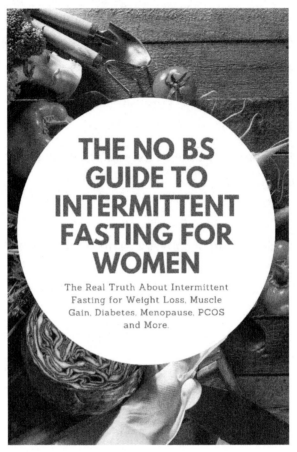

IGOR KLIBANOV

The No BS Guide to Intermittent Fasting for Women: The Real Truth About Intermittent Fasting for Weight Loss, Muscle Gain, Diabetes, Menopause, PCOS and More.

Are you looking for an honest, no BS intermittent fasting guide? There is a lot of hype and dishonest information about intermittent fasting. But is it all it's cracked up to be? In this book, get an unbiased evidence-based look at where intermittent fasting really shines, where it falls short of the claims, and where it's harmful.

You can expect to learn:

- Intermittent fasting for women over 50/intermittent fasting for menopause: is it as effective as in younger women?

- Intermittent fasting for PCOS: does it improve insulin, testosterone and estrogen in these women?

- Intermittent fasting for diabetes: the conditions that it must meet in order to lower both blood sugar and insulin levels.

- Intermittent fasting for weight loss: how does it compare to a regular calorie distribution?

- Intermittent fasting for muscle gain: is it more or less effective than a more traditional approach?

- Additional chapters on intermittent fasting for heart health, bone health (osteoporosis) and PMS.

If you want to pick up a copy, you can go to **https://amzn.to/48qnbL7**.

Services Offered by the Author

Personal Training and Nutritional Consulting

If you're in or around the Greater Toronto Area, you can see whether you qualify to train with the author, or one of his team members.

The training starts with an initial assessment, where the author learns about you and your goals, injuries, medical conditions, medications, and more.

After the initial assessment, the author crafts an exercise and nutrition program made to fit you like a finely-tailored suit.

As you continue making progress, adjustments will be made to your program, to make sure you're moving closer and closer to your goal.

If you'd like to see whether this is right for you, simply email Igor@TorontoFitnessOnline.com.

Online Coaching

If you're outside the Greater Toronto Area, but want to benefit from professional expertise, the author has specifically trained a hand-picked, elite team of fitness professionals to train clients remotely.

The online coaching starts with an initial assessment, where your coach learns about you and your goals, injuries, medical conditions, medications, and more.

After that, an exercise and/or nutrition program will be crafted to fit your goals, your body, your time and equipment availability.

Adjustments to the program will be made on a regular basis, to keep you progressing.

If you'd like to see whether this is right for you, simply email

Igor@TorontoFitnessOnline.com.

Consulting

If you don't need a program made for you, but you just have questions to ask, and you're reconfused by all the information out there, so you just want the highest-quality, most accurate information handed to you on a silver platter, we can do that.

You'll save tons of time and frustration on the research and trial and error it takes to figure out what works for you.

If you'd like to see whether this is right for you, simply email

Igor@TorontoFitnessOnline.com.

Public Speaking

Igor Klibanov is one of the most sought-after wellness speakers in the Greater Toronto Area, having delivered over 400 speaking engagements (at the time of this writing) to some of Canada's largest corporations, including the Royal Bank of Canada, IBM, Bosch, and many others.

Topics include:

1. STOP EXERCISING! The Way You Are Doing it Now

2. Exercise and Nutrition for Mental Health

3. 8 Hidden Reasons You Can't Lose Weight

4. Everything You Wanted to Know About Nutritional Supplements, But Were Afraid to Ask

5. No Pain, All Gain: How to Exercise the Right Way for YOUR Chronic Condition

6. Exercise for Different Body Types

7. Fitness for Females

8. Weight Loss for Women Over 40

9. End Emotional Eating

10. Healthy Food That Poisons: Why You're Getting Sicker and Fatter Despite Eating Healthier

11. How to Get a Flat Stomach, Round Butt and Lose Weight

12. How to Prevent Neck Pain and Lower Back Pain

13. Running for Non-Runners

14. Stand Up Straight. A 4-Step Approach to Fixing Your Posture

15. How to Double Your Testosterone Naturally in 6 Months

16. How to lose 10, 20, 50 or more pounds without crash dieting

17. Stress Management for the Busy Professional

18. How to Change Your Mind to Change Your Body

19. Fitness over 50

20. A New Model of Pain

21. Workshop: Exercise progressions and Regressions

22. Workshop: Self tissue release

To book Igor for a speaking engagement, email Igor@TorontoFitnessOnline.com.

Printed in Great Britain
by Amazon

40517669R00119